PREPARING FOR THE
ANESTHESIA ORALS

BOARD STIFF

PREPARING FOR THE
ANESTHESIA ORALS

BOARD STIFF

CHRISTOPHER J. GALLAGHER, MD

ASSISTANT PROFESSOR OF ANESTHESIOLOGY
DUKE UNIVERSITY SCHOOL OF MEDICINE
DURHAM, NORTH CAROLINA

DAVID A. LUBARSKY, MD

ASSISTANT PROFESSOR OF ANESTHESIOLOGY
DUKE UNIVERSITY SCHOOL OF MEDICINE
DURHAM, NORTH CAROLINA

BUTTERWORTH–HEINEMANN
BOSTON LONDON SINGAPORE SYDNEY TORONTO WELLINGTON

Every effort has been made to ensure that the drug dosage schedules within this text are accurate and conform to standards accepted at time of publication. However, as treatment recommendations vary in the light of continuing research and clinical experience, the reader is advised to verify drug dosage schedules herein with information found on product information sheets. This is especially true in cases of new or infrequently used drugs.

Library of Congress Cataloging-in-Publication Data

Gallagher, Christopher J.
    Preparing for the anesthesia orals : board stiff /
Christopher J. Gallagher, David A. Lubarsky.
      p. cm.
    Includes index.
    ISBN 0-7506-9240-5 (previously ISBN 0-409-90207-1)
    1. Anesthesia—Examinations, questions, etc.
I. Lubarsky, David A. II. Title.
    [DNLM: 1.Anesthesia—examination questions.
WO 218 G162p]
RD82.3.G35 1990
617.9′6′076—dc20
DNLM/DLC
for Library of Congress   89-9820

British Library Cataloguing in Publication Data
Gallagher, Chris
    Preparing for the anaesthesia orals: board stiff.
    1. Medicine. Anaesthesia. Questions & answers
I. Title II. Lubarsky, David
617′.96′076

ISBN 0-7506-9240-5 (previously ISBN 0-409-90207-1)

Butterworth–Heinemann   10 9 8 7
80 Montvale Avenue
Stoneham, MA 02180   Printed in the United States of America

CONTENTS

Preface   *vii*

1   What You're In For   *1*

2   What to Read   *3*

3   Horror Stories   *5*

4   Encouraging Stories   *7*

5   What the Exam Is   *9*

6   What the Exam Isn't   *11*

7   Vital Signs Are Vital   *13*

8   The Machine Age   *17*

9   Putting on Airs   *23*

10   The Heart Is a Lonely Hunter   *25*

11   Airway, Airway, Who Lost the Airway?   *29*

12   Traumaland   *33*

13   Watersports   *35*

14   I Don't Know Nuthin' 'bout Birthin' No Babies, Miz Scarlett   *37*

15   Little Rascals   *41*

16 Rockin' Round the Block   *47*

17 The Eyes Have It   *49*

18 Pâté   *51*

19 Colloid Is Thicker than Water   *53*

20 Sydney Greenstreet Plays the Fat Man   *55*

21 Sample Questions   *57*

22 Grab Bag Questions   *175*

23 Grab Bag Answers   *179*

24 A Note on Dress and Conduct   *187*

25 Post Mortem   *189*

Glossary   *191*

Index   *193*

PREFACE

In the beginning, there was half the big syringe, all the small syringe. Then came fentanyl, somatosensory evoked potentials, halothane hepatitis, and a host of other afflictions to vex the spirit of the average oral board examinee. Where to turn? The literature? Go ahead, open the last 17 volumes of *Anesthesiology*. Do you really care what happens to slices of salamander fetal hippocampus when exposed to the latest benzodiazepine antagonist? Are you about to try to disprove the findings yourself? Wrong, bucko. The questions that bother you are much more mundane—and more important.

Soon you'll be staring down the glare of two examiners who have forgotten more in the last 15 minutes than you've learned in your whole wretched lifetime. They aren't concerned with what happens in the achondroplastic dwarf on phenelzine who just aspirated a peanut and has had no IV access ever since a 99% burn. They want to know whether you'll cancel a generic case for a generically high blood pressure. Try to find the answer! Look long and hard. Read all the textbooks. Direct answers are hard to find!

Devoid of any national renown, the two of us have taken it on ourselves to distill the essence of the oral boards into a small, portable study guide. Academicians in the field of anesthesiology may cringe at the thought that this book is even associated with their discipline—the authors are the types you see at a meeting, not presenting abstracts, but hanging out at the pool demanding piña coladas for breakfast.

We have invented a large variety of oral board scenarios and present them step by step. To develop these questions, we culled information from scores of examinees. We talked to many who passed and a few who flunked. From the recurrent themes that appeared year after year, we invented questions similar to those encountered on the oral boards.

- No examiners were approached about specific questions.
- No examiners were connected in any way to the production of this book.

- These questions are meant to resemble oral board questions. Any verbatim reproduction of an actual board question is coincidental.

We have not annotated every fact in this book. We did that for three reasons. First, this is a review, a guide book. If you need a ton of references, then consult the heavily referenced textbooks. Second, most people in their last few weeks of preparation for the boards don't look up a lot of original articles. Third,[1] when[2-4] you're[5] reading (Rumpelstiltskin, 1856) through[ibid] a[4,6,7,8] review (Jumpinjohosephrat, 1977), the flow gets a little choppy if every other word is coated with superscripts and references.

This book will provide you with answers to those tough "there's no right answer" questions. Maybe not *the* answer, but an answer you can defend. We stick our necks out on a variety of complex and controversial questions. We discuss difficult cases where you must balance the anesthetic considerations for two or more organ systems concomitantly. We show you how to make a rational decision that you should be able to defend. Making rational decisions that you can defend should get you through the boards.

Good luck!

C.J.G.
D.A.L.

1 | WHAT YOU'RE IN FOR

Chances are good that the two people sitting across the table from you will be a little smarter than you. Nonetheless, a knowledge of what their job is will enable you to prepare better for your hour of agony.

Board certification in any specialty is a testament to the fact that a group of peers have reviewed your performance and found you to be qualified as a consultant in the field. The American Board of Anesthesiology does just that. Through their written and oral examination, they assess whether or not you should be called a consultant in anesthesiology. If this certification were easy to get, it would not represent much of anything. Thus, it should come as no surprise that the examiners are not going to ask what your favorite color is. What, then, will they ask you?

Reasonable questions. However, these same reasonable questions are also virtually unanswerable unless you've thought about your responses beforehand. There aren't necessarily absolute right and wrong responses, just logical and consistent ones. These are everyday questions of judgment: getting further preoperative evaluation, canceling a case, deciding the extent of monitoring, and knowing when to pick a fight with the "give 'em a little whiff of gas" surgeon. Having an organized approach to the preoperative, intraoperative, and postoperative assessment and management of critical organ pathophysiology is hard to do. To communicate that orally without stumbling over your own words is harder than reciting "Peter Piper picked a peck of pickled peppers."

Now, anyone who has recited tongue twisters and nursery rhymes knows that if you do them enough times, you can say them in your sleep. Practice makes perfect. So it goes with preparation for the oral exams. The more you practice giving organized responses out loud, the better you will do. Talk to the mirror, practice with your colleagues, force your spouse to listen to your practice answers, tell your dog. If you can't explain your reasoning out loud before the test, you won't be able to do it during the test.

You will be graded on your responses in the following categories: judgment, application, adaptability, clarity. *Judgment* means treating the patient appropriately—like giving ketamine rather than 750 mg of pentothal to a trauma patient. *Application* deals with the way you use your knowledge to analyze the anesthetic considerations for a complex case. *Adaptability* means the examiners are going to manipulate the case so that whatever you want to do (a regional) will not work and you will quickly have to formulate an alternative plan (a general anesthetic). Adaptability will also be tested during the "unforeseen" (unless you've read this book) life-threatening complications that inevitably will accompany the execution of even a perfectly reasonable anesthetic plan. Facts themselves are not a grading consideration. You need facts to judge, apply, and adapt, but your fate on the exam does not rest on specific nit-picking details. *Clarity* is all-important. Before you answer the examiners' questions, make sure you are answering what they are asking. Take a deep breath, organize your thoughts, and address the pertinent points. We have heard of too many smart people ruining their exam by being asked to count to five and responding with a discourse on the relationships of sequential prime numbers. They exasperate the examiners and waste precious moments of their half hour.

Suppose your resident or nurse anesthetist asks you to explain the special considerations in anesthetizing a patient with thyroid dysfunction. If you find yourself tripping over your words and ideas, go home, read about it, return to work, and give that resident or nurse anesthetist an organized lecture on the topic. Your colleague will be amazed, and you will be prepared. Best of all, practicing like this will organize your thinking and make you a more effective clinician. That, perhaps, is the most rewarding aspect of preparing for the boards. Both authors found that their ability to give didactic instruction to residents improved dramatically while preparing for the exam.

2 | WHAT TO READ

Everything helps, nothing hurts. The more you read, the smarter you'll be. What to focus on, though, if you're too busy to go over Miller, Stoelting, and Goodman and Gilman? Basic texts and reviews have a lot more information in them than you usually give them credit for. No doubt you've leafed through Baby Miller (the short version of the textbook) a few times and kind of skimmed the text, figuring you would read a real text to get real meat. But look closely at the section on pulmonary function tests, for example. The indications in Baby Miller for who needs PFTs and who doesn't are as good as any other list of indications. If you memorize that list and have it at your fingertips, you'll be as capable as anyone. Other sources of basic information are equally as valuable. The Mass. General handbook is second to none for useful tidbits like maximum doses of local anesthetics, indications for preop tests, and the protocol for malignant hyperthermia. It also has the distinct advantage that it's easy to lug around in case you want to look something over while you're at the beach or on the bus (for you New Yorkers). Read the basic stuff over and over again. The basic stuff is what the examiners will focus on and what you will curse yourself for having neglected.

Since you know the patients you will see on the exam will be very complex, you can be sure they will have coexisting diseases. Sound familiar? You've got it, Stoelting's *Anesthesia and Co-existing Disease* was our personal favorite while studying for this test. Short on time? At least review the sections titled "Anesthetic Considerations" so you don't overlook something obvious or give a patently ridiculous drug.

How about the ASA refresher courses? Purists point out that these courses are not peer-reviewed and say you shouldn't actually read them—or at least you shouldn't admit it in stylish company. We disagree. The refresher courses are given by a high-powered bunch of people who are up on the latest. For example, recommendations on dantrolene seem to change every year, so getting the latest word from a world-renowned expert will put you in good shape for the orals.

Best of all, practice a few oral exams with someone, identify where you're stumbling, then read up on that specific topic.

Recommended Reading

Dorsch JA, Dorsch SE. *Understanding Anesthesia Equipment,* 2d edition. Baltimore: Williams & Wilkins, 1984.

Firestone LL et al. *Clinical Anesthesia Procedures of the Massachusetts General Hospital,* 3d edition. Boston: Little, Brown, 1988.

Miller RD (ed). *Anesthesia,* 2d edition. New York: Churchill Livingstone, 1986.

Stoelting RK, Dierdorf SF, McCammon R. *Anesthesia and Co-existing Disease,* 2d edition. New York: Churchill Livingstone, 1988.

Stoelting RK, Miller RD. *Basics of Anesthesia,* 2d edition. New York: Churchill Livingstone, 1989.

3 | HORROR STORIES

Everyone knows someone smart who flunked. The one question they answered wrong, the one absolutely fatal recommendation, or the one really nasty examiner who was out to get them was cited as the cause of the downfall. Was that really the reason?

Having discussed this somewhat delicate topic with a number of people, we found one recurrent theme. Those who failed tended to get rattled early in the exam and never got back on track. For example, one candidate was asked, "What are the anesthetic implications of acromegaly?" He became completely unglued and could not think of a single thing. For the rest of the exam he kept thinking back to that question and didn't concentrate on subsequent questions. At no point did he take charge of the exam. He was playing "catch-up ball," so to speak.

Another examinee was pinned to the wall on some equipment-related questions early in the exam. Shaken by these questions, he too couldn't get back on track.

What is the take-home lesson? No *one* question will sink you, but letting one question rattle you to the bone may keep you from taking command of the exam. You have 30 minutes to show these examiners you know something, and floundering does not impress them.

How do you bail out? There is no harm in saying, "I don't know, can we move on to another topic?" Better that than burning up precious minutes going around in circles. The examiners will most likely oblige you at least once during the exam—just don't make that a mainstay of your exam strategy.

How about some good news to counter all those horror stories? If you stick with the system, even if it takes three tries, you stand a better than 90% chance of passing the exam eventually. So even if you fall by the wayside on the first attempt, life is not over, the sun will still shine, your friends will still talk to you at parties, and you most likely will pass.

4 | ENCOURAGING STORIES

Everyone knows someone with the intelligence of a newt who passed the exam.

5 | WHAT THE EXAM IS

When you get your packet from the ABA, it will have a practice exam in it. *Read it carefully!* That practice exam details the exact way you will be examined. Gear your studying and your practice oral presentations to that pattern. In each of the two rooms that you will be examined in, there will be a short, three-sentence stem question. You will be asked 5 minutes of preop questions, approximately 10 minutes of intraop questions, and 5 minutes of postop questions. In each room, the last part of the exam will be a few grab-bag questions designed to cover areas of anesthesia that the stem question has not touched on.

With every patient, we puzzle over the optimal preop assessment and how to manage intraop and postop complications. An oral exam is just a way of saying aloud what we do every day.

When taking the exam, mentally place yourself in your daily workplace. For example, when they ask you what to do if the patient gets cyanotic, put yourself in your favorite room and go through the steps you normally take when your patient's oxygen saturation drops. This takes the question from the spooky realm of the abstract to the reassuringly concrete. Then you need only recreate the management of a routine intraoperative complication.

6 | WHAT THE EXAM ISN'T

The examiners are not evil people bent on the destruction of your life's ambitions. They are board-certified anesthesiologists interested in getting you board certified. They have no absolute quota to fill, no curve to adhere to, and, surprisingly, they may have no better answers than you to the hard questions. They merely have the luxury of asking the hard questions and waiting for you to answer.

Nor is the exam a witch hunt. If you are fishing for the answer, they will sometimes give you a little prompting to get you going. For example, on Chris's exam he was missing the boat on a reference to the oculocardiac reflex. His examiner said, "Now the pulse *has* dropped to 70." He grabbed that safety line and pulled himself back into the examiners' good graces.

The exam is not exactly a pleasant conversation with encouraging interchange. The most unnerving aspect is the lack of feedback. You do not always get hints. It's worth practicing several exams with a stone-faced person. Your friend asks a question and, instead of giving a nice "OK" or "that's what I would do," cuts you off in midsentence and goes on to the next question. You'll sit there wondering, "Did I just kill the patient? Would it have been better to use a Swan?" and you'll have some notion of what the real exam will feel like. During the real exam, you plod along and endure an existential angst.

At the end of the stem question there will be some vital signs and maybe one lab value. *Pay attention* to these—they are there for a purpose. If the hematocrit is up, there must be a reason (chronic hypoxemia, heart disease). If the heart rate is up, it is up for a reason (arrhythmia, hypovolemia, pain). Vital signs are vital.

Groom yourself to handle every aberration in vital signs. In fact, that is the essence of an anesthesiologist's job. In the intraoperative part of the oral examination, you will probably have to handle at least two aberrations in vital signs. Work on a good systematic response to each of the following:

- Hypertension
- Hypotension
- Tachycardia
- Bradycardia
- Hypoxemia
- Hypercapnia

You probably have a fairly good response to these right now, but it should be practiced *aloud* again and again and again. Until you're sick of it. Until your mouth has achieved muscle memory from forming the phrases so often.

"The patient's heart rate goes from 70 to 120."

First a mushy response, then an organized one:

Well, uh, what's the blood pressure? Well, then it could be, is the vaporizer on? It could be from pain. You want to be sure the oxygen is on, is the incentive, no, I mean is the oxygen analyzer on? He could be in, what's the ECG show?

It takes no Einstein to recognize that Marvin Mushmouth's response to the question is not going to win any trips to Stockholm. Sammy Slick gives a more systematic approach to the same question:

"Tachycardia can be either primary or secondary."

A. Primary tachycardia—from pathology inherent to the heart
   1. Supraventricular arrhythmia
   2. Ventricular arrhythmia
B. Secondary tachycardia—from sympathetic stimulation
   1. Hypoxemia
      "This is life-threatening, I would always address it first." [If you don't say it, they don't know that you know it.]
   2. Hypercapnia
   3. Decreased oxygen delivery
      a. Anemia
      b. Decreased cardiac output
   4. Pain (probably associated with hypertension)
      a. Somatic (surgical stimuli)
      b. Visceral (distended bladder)
      c. Sympathetic (tourniquet pain)
   5. Hypovolemia (probably associated with hypotension)
      a. Absolute (dehydration, hemorrhage)
      b. Relative (tamponade, pneumothorax, PEEP)
         "Much less likely causes of this tachycardia include an inotrope running in too fast, or the remote possibility of pheochromocytoma or carcinoid syndrome."

Sammy Slick's answer is systematic. Although it doesn't list every possible cause of tachycardia, it does hit the major ones. Most important, this approach focuses on ABC—airway, breathing, circulation—that is, it looks at hypoxemia and hypercapnia. As in the OR, you must first and foremost *assure adequacy of ventilation.*

Always say you will check your ventilation first at the first sign of trouble. You do so in the OR, don't you? (If you don't, it's high time you did.)

The approach to hypertension is similar to the approach to tachycardia, that is, consider primary hypertension and then consider hypertension secondary to sympathetic stimulation. Can hypoxemia or hypercapnia cause hypertension? Yes, so *first check the adequacy of ventilation.*

For hypoxemia, take a geographic approach.

A. Wall to endotracheal tube—go from the wall to the ET tube to cover mechanical causes for decreased oxygen delivery:
   1. Wrong composition of gas delivered—low inspired oxygen or pipeline crossover

2. No gas delivery—disconnect, ventilator turned off, or the switch used to change from manual to mechanical ventilation on the newer machines is in the wrong position

B. Endotracheal tube to lungs
1. Endobronchial or esophageal intubation
2. Kink or clog
3. Disconnect

C. Thorax, outermost to innermost
1. Chest wall/diaphragm
   a. Hypoventilation from weakness due to residual neuromuscular blockade
   b. Kyphoscoliosis, flail chest, phrenic nerve damage
2. Pleura—pneumo-, hydro-, hemo-, or chylothorax
3. Lung parenchyma—aspiration, pneumonia, atelectasis, ventilation-perfusion (V/Q) mismatch from patient positioning or from one-lung anesthesia
4. Pulmonary vasculature
   a. Emboli, thrombi, fat, amniotic fluid
   b. Right-to-left intrapulmonary shunts
5. Heart
   a. Cardiac failure
   b. Right-to-left intracardiac shunts
6. CNS
   a. Apnea from narcotics or inhaled anesthetics
   b. Damage to the respiratory center

There are other causes of hypoxemia, but the approach just outlined is a systematic rundown of the major causes you would not want to miss. *From the wall to the machine to the tubing to the ET tube to the lungs. From the chest wall to the pleura to the parenchyma to the pulmonary vasculature, then out to the heart and the brain.* The specific examples will come easily if you do the differential the same way every day. Even if you don't hit each specific cause, if you show the examiners that you're approaching the problem in a slick way, they will cut you a lot more slack.

Hypercapnia will appear without fail. Be systematic: first give the major categories, then elaborate on the specific reasons for hypercapnia under each category. The CO_2 is up because the patient is making too much CO_2, or breathing in CO_2, or eliminating too little CO_2.

A. Overproduction of CO_2
1. Malignant hyperthermia
2. Thyrotoxicosis
3. Sepsis
B. Decreased elimination
1. Hypoventilation
    a. Neuromuscular blockade
    b. Inhaled or IV anesthetic agent
    c. Inappropriate ventilator settings
2. Bronchospasm
3. Esophageal intubation (unlikely to present just as hypercapnia)
C. Rebreathing
1. Exhausted CO_2 reabsorber
2. Malfunctioning one-way valves in a circle system
3. Low gas flows with Mapleson-type circuits

This systematic approach to hypercapnia—first hitting the major categories then elucidating the individual causes—will satisfy your examiners.

The final vital sign you must prepare for is bradycardia. Approach it as you did tachycardia, considering the primary and the secondary causes.

A. Primary
1. Sick sinus syndrome
2. Complete heart block
B. Secondary
1. Drug-induced
    a. Atrial fibrillation with excess digoxin (vagotonic)
    b. Narcotics and neuromuscular blockers (vagotonic)
    c. Beta-blockers (sympatholysis)
    d. Calcium channel blockers
    e. Halothane depression of sinoatrial node
2. Vagal stimulation
    a. Oculocardiac reflex
    b. Traction on the peritoneum
    c. Laryngoscopy
    d. Baroreceptor reflex

Using this primary/secondary approach will organize your thinking and prevent you from missing a major cause of bradycardia.

Vital signs are vital.

Preparing for the Anesthesia Orals

"God forbid they should ask me to draw a line isolation monitor!"

Sound familiar? Ever actually tried to draw one? How about all that other equipment we struggle with every day? What kind of relief valves are on the scavenging system? If these kinds of questions make you lose all libido, if they wake you up in the middle of the night, then we have bad news for you: you've got to sit down and have a go at Dorsch & Dorsch. Anyone who has read that quaint and curious volume of forgotten lore will tell you that it is dry. It is real dry. We are talking *dry*. Sahara, Mojave, Sinai, Dorsch & Dorsch.

But it is good.

Concentrate on learning what you really should know to run a safe anesthetic: how vaporizers work, the advantages of different breathing circuits, and safety factors on the anesthesia machine.

Vaporizers work by one of two simple designs: bubble through or flow over. Either the carrier oxygen is sent directly through the anesthetic liquid (bubble through) or the carrier oxygen flows over the liquid anesthetic (flow over). Some examinees have been asked to draw a vaporizer. A *simplified* diagram follows that should suffice for the exam (Figure 1). The examiners are not interested in a complete, detailed sketch that shows every nut and bolt. They want you to know the principles of the machines we use every day.

Different breathing circuits have different advantages. There are only a few facts that merit your consideration. If you are familiar with the alphabet soup of the Mapleson classification, then you really should be pursuing a career in protons, photons, and quarks. The simplified approach to this confusing topic lies in memorizing aspects of those circuits that you might use in your practice and ignoring the rest.

There are four types of breathing circuits:

A. Open—open drop technique such as ether
B. Semi-open
    1. The Mapleson menagerie

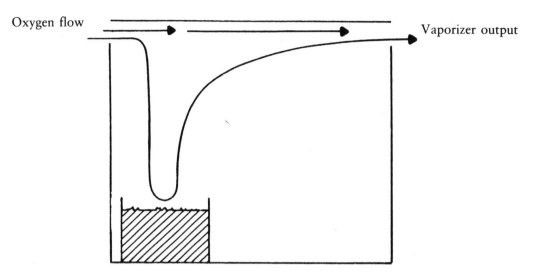

Oxygen flow

Vaporizer output

Figure 1
A vaporizer. Some of the oxygen flowing into the vaporizer passes over (or through) the anesthetic liquid and some bypasses it. The anesthetic liquid is represented by the shaded area.

    2. Jackson Reese, a modified Mapleson E
    3. Bain, a modified Mapleson D
C. Semiclosed—your generic circle system used in the OR every day
D. Closed—your circle with the pop-off valve closed

Each circuit has its advantages:

A. Open
    1. Lightweight, portable, useful in the field of battle
    2. No complex equipment is needed
    3. Useful in situations of extreme need, such as in poor countries
B. Semi-open
    1. Lightweight, portable, and disposable
    2. There are no valves, so resistance is low
C. Semiclosed
    1. Rebreathing is possible, therefore heat is conserved
    2. A CO_2 absorber is employed so CO_2 rebreathing is avoided, even at low flow rates
D. Closed
    1. Heat and anesthetic agent are conserved
    2. Saves money
    3. Good teaching guide for understanding uptake and distribution

The most commonly used circuits merit separate consideration.

Mapleson D and *Jackson Reese* (a modification of Mapleson E) are lightweight and portable. They allow you to be in close proximity to your pediatric patient. Since they do not utilize one-way valves, they have a low resistance to breathing. The force necessary to open a unidirectional flow valve is substantial for the pediatric patient. Both these circuits allow spontaneous and controlled respiratory patterns without significant re-breathing as long as high gas flows (about 2.5 × minute ventilation) are used.

The *Bain* is a modified Mapleson D. All the benefits listed above apply to the Bain. The co-axial fresh gas inflow conserves heat but may lead to unnoticed fresh gas disconnects and rebreathing.

The *circle system* conserves heat and humidity (low flows, absorber) and the rebreathing allows decreased anesthetic gas consumption. The unidirectional valves in the circle system make the resistance to breathing unacceptable for patients under 10 kg.

"What safety factors are present on the anesthesia machine?" has appeared on oral exams. "In particular, what safety factors pertaining to oxygen delivery are present?"

Safety factors are built into the connections, the machine itself, the ventilator, and the breathing circuit:

A. Wall to inlet
   1. Diameter-indexed safety system, which couples oxygen and nitrous oxide to the wall
   2. Colored tubing
   3. Pin-index safety system, which couples the cylinders to the machine
   4. Colored cylinders
B. The machine
   1. Fluted control handle for oxygen rotameter
   2. Oxygen located on the far right side of the manifold (so that a break in the manifold is least likely to produce a hypoxic gas mixture, i.e., a crack would leak N_2O or an N_2O-O_2 mixture depending on the position of the crack, but never O_2 alone)
   3. Stopper located on top of flowmeters so that the indicator ball/bobbin won't plug the manifold
   4. Fail-safe mechanism that alarms if oxygen pressure is below 25 lb/sq. in. *The fail-safe mechanism does not guarantee oxygen flow, only oxygen pressure*
   5. Oxygen ratio monitor controller to link N_2O flow to oxygen flow

C. The ventilator
   1. Disconnect alarm indicating low pressure. *The ventilator may disconnect and the tubing may press against the drapes, so the ventilator will continue to cycle while the patient dies*
   2. Alarms for subatmospheric, continuing, and high pressure
   3. Oxygen powering the bellows so that a hole in the bellows will let pure oxygen enter
D. The breathing circuit
   Oxygen analyzer. *Mandatory equipment—there is no way of knowing that you are delivering oxygen unless there is an oxygen analyzer*

Things misfire on the anesthesia machine. A few problems typical of those asked on the oral board exam follow.

1. The oxygen is on 2 L, the nitrous is on 2 L, the patient is on the ventilator, and the FIO_2 reads 85%.
   Answer: Oxygen powers the bellows. There is a hole in the bellows and O_2 is entering the bellows, yielding a higher FIO_2.
2. The reservoir bag keeps collapsing despite high gas flows.
   Answer: The scavenging system is sucking too hard and pulling gases out of the circle system.
3. The reservoir bag keeps inflating despite low gas flows.
   Answer: The scavenging system is clogged or the pop-off valve isn't working.
4. Oxygen flowmeter reads 5 L, N_2O is 0 L, but the FIO_2 reads 21%.
   Answer: Pipeline crossover or wrong cylinder forced into the oxygen yoke. Probably air is being used rather than oxygen.
5. A cylinder is hanging crooked and is hissing.
   Answer: The cylinder is improperly connected or the wrong cylinder is in the yoke.
6. The oxygen knob is turned off but the rotameter reads 5 L.
   Answer: There is dust in the flowmeter, making the bobbin stick.
7. The ventilator is cycling and no alarm is sounding, but the chest is not moving.
   Answer: The alarm has not been turned off. The ventilator hose is pressing against the drapes, so the low-pressure alarm is not going off.
8. The ventilator does not fill.
   Answer: A disconnect somewhere in the system. If you look all over and can't find the site, hand ventilate with an Ambu bag and a separate oxygen cylinder.

9. Oxygen flow is 5 L, nitrous flow is 5 L, FIO$_2$ reads 26% and the ventilator is cycling.

   Answer: Hanging bellows is drawing in room air from a partial disconnect in any part of the circuit. No, we didn't mention the archaic hanging bellows, but neither may the examiners.

10. Capnogram shows inspired CO$_2$.

    Answer: One-way valve malfunctions and causes rebreathing or else the CO$_2$ absorber is exhausted. Channeling through the absorber may have the same effect.

Electrical safety is not as forbidding as you might think. You do need to draw the circuits to get them down. Keep in mind that to have a shock hazard, you must complete a circuit. No circuit, no shock. Circuit complete: possible shock (Figure 2).

A question often asked is, "What do you do if the line isolation monitor goes off?" The patient is at risk for a macroshock; the alarm is going off. You have to find the machine at fault and stop that damned buzzing. If the line isolation monitor alarms *before* the patient is brought into the OR, you must postpone or move the case. If the alarm sounds *during* the case, then unplug the appliances in your room one by one, starting with the last one you turned on, until you find out which machine is improperly grounded.

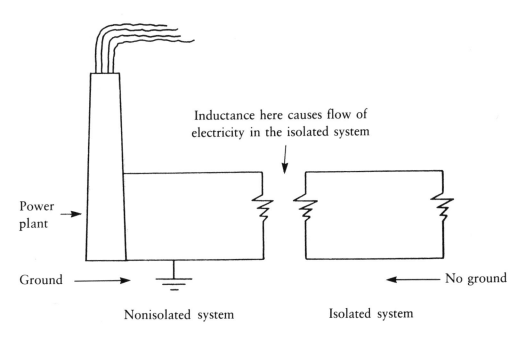

Figure 2
An isolated electrical system. The line isolation monitor alarms if the isolated (that is, non-grounded) system acts as if it were grounded.

Micro or macroshock? Watch the decimal points. Ventricular fibrillation from a current applied directly to the heart can occur at 50 *micro*-amps. Microshock can occur when an ECG machine that has not been cleared by biomedical engineering is connected to a pacer wire or fluid-filled CVP catheter. Any patient with a central line in place is never truly safe from a microshock. (Spooky, isn't it? Makes you wonder about the advisability of having that ungrounded compact disk player sitting on top of your pulse oximeter.)

The threshold for the line isolation monitor alarm is 2 *milli*amps. When the alarm sounds, you have completed a circuit with *at least* 2 milliamps of current flowing—you could have a zillion. That puts the patient at risk for ventricular fibrillation, which can occur when a current of 100 *milli*amps is applied to the body.

Don't let a fear of electrical safety questions make your hair stand on end.

Pulmonary function tests always appear on the oral boards. Always. Be crystal clear and concise when asking for PFTs in the preoperative evaluation of a patient with lung disease. Any patient who is symptomatic (non-cardiogenic dyspnea, chronic cough with purulent sputum production and a smoking history) or who has been treated chronically with bronchodilator therapy for severe COPD or asthma, or who is undergoing lung resection needs PFTs. The examiner asks, "Which ones and why?" The usual Marvin Mushmouth error is, "Well, you know, all of them, you know, the PFTs you always get." Wrong! That answer shows the examiners that you are not thinking, you are just reacting like an automaton. A Sammy Slick answer, one that shows you have *thought* abut the PFTs, is "FEV_1, FVC, maximal expiratory flow rate (MEFR), and maximum mid-expiratory flow (MMEF) 25–75%. These will allow me to assess the presence of obstructive versus restrictive disease (FEV_1/FVC), the large airways obstruction associated with asthma (MEFR), and give me an effort-independent evaluation of small airways disease (MMEF)." Clear, concise, thoughtful.

Draw a baseline blood gas and evaluate PFTs post bronchodilator therapy to see if improvement occurs. Then you can answer the examiner's question, "Will you do this case? If not, how long will you wait?" You respond, "Patients with abnormal PFTs are at increased risk for postoperative pulmonary complications. Treatment for 48 to 72 hours preoperatively to maximize their medical management (with IV aminophylline, inhaled beta-agonists, stopping smoking, preoperative instruction in incentive spirometry, and possibly steroids) will decrease their operative risk." Such snappy responses mark you as a consultant.

When a lobectomy is planned, anticipate the possibility of a pneumonectomy secondary to a vascular catastrophe or a more extensive tumor than expected. Therefore, the patient always must be prepared for an entire pneumonectomy. Ascertain that the patient will not be permanently ventilator dependent following resection of an entire lung. If certain PFT criteria are not met, then order split lung function studies. These criteria are listed in Table 1.

TABLE 1. *Preoperative Pulmonary Function Tests and Operative Risk of Pneumonectomy*

Testing Phase	PFT[a]	Increased Operative Risk Result
Whole lung tests	Arterial blood gases	Hypercapnia on room air
	Spirometry	FEV_1 <50% of FVC
		FEV_1 <2 L
		MBC <50% predicted
	Lung volume	RV/TLC >50%
Single lung tests	Right–left (individual lung) split-function tests	Predicted postoperative FEV_1 <0.85 L or >70% blood flow to diseased lung
Mimic postop condition	Temporary unilateral occlusion of main pulmonary artery	Mean pulmonary artery pressure increase >30 to 40 mm Hg

[a]The testing phases and PFT are listed in order of proper temporal performance and increasing invasiveness.

RV = residual volume; TLC = total lung capacity; MBC = maximum breathing capacity.

Source: Benumof JL, Alfery DD. Anesthesia for thoracic surgery. In Miller RD (ed), Anesthesia, 2d edition. New York: Churchill Livingstone, 1986:1373.

The criteria themselves are not so important as knowing that they exist. That is, even if you forget the 50% figures, for example, you could say, "Although the exact numbers escape me, I would order split function lung studies, if necessary, to make sure that the patient could tolerate a pneumonectomy. The goal of those studies is to answer the question, 'Can this patient undergo a planned or unplanned pneumonectomy and remain ventilator independent?" For a planned lobectomy where you expect the patient to be unable to tolerate a pneumonectomy, the decision to proceed can be turned over to the surgeon and patient by informing them of and discussing the risk of operating.

The examiners will grade you on your thinking, not on your memorizing.

10 | THE HEART IS A LONELY HUNTER

Alan Arkin played the role of a deaf mute in this stirring movie. He expressed the inexpressible and yet never opened his mouth. You will have no such luxury. The toughest questions refer to the preop workup of patients with cardiac disease. The "definitive" suggestions you are about to read are controversial. But somebody has to put his neck on the chopping block. The famous authors of the other texts won't, and we will. That's why you bought this book.

The killer on the boards is, "What preop evaluation do you want in this patient?"

"Well, er, ideally you would have a cath, but do you *insist* on a cath, and, um, well, a MUGA would be good, but then again, I wouldn't really insist on it." Well what in blazes *do* you insist on? All those cardiac studies! (If you wouldn't order a MUGA because you can't remember what it is, the acronym stands for *multiple uptake gated acquisition scan*. The glossary at the end contains the abbreviations used throughout this book.)

As if the welter of cardiac studies were not enough, how about the stream of patients who *just might* have cardiac disease: the long-time smoker who gets short of breath easily, the carotid endarterectomy patient, the femoropopliteal bypass veteran?

To start sorting out this complicated workup, get as much free information as possible. If the patient already has a cath, read it. Compare the preop ECG to an old ECG. Get a chest x-ray and compare it to an old chest x-ray. Squeeze that history and physical for all they are worth. Determine the answer to:

1. Is the pattern of angina unstable (new angina, change in pattern, angina at rest)? If the angina is unstable, the patient is not a candidate for elective surgery and needs a cardiology workup. The extent of the cardiology workup is determined by the cardiologist.

2. Does the patient have congestive heart failure? If so, she is not a candidate for an elective procedure until her condition is deemed optimal as determined by the cardiologist.

Don't go to the big-time invasive tests until you *really* have every ounce of information from the noninvasive data. Emphasize *clarity* and *purpose* for each test you order: "I want an ECG to determine if the patient has had a previous myocardial infarction and to see if the patient is in atrial fibrillation" versus "Gee, Wally, we better get an ECG, huh?"

Let's look at those catch-22's from a few paragraphs back. First, the smoker who gets short of breath. Is the patient's shortness of breath cardiac, pulmonary, or both cardiac and pulmonary in origin? Get what you can get for "free"—ECG, old chest x-ray, history, and physical. What if you can't differentiate between pulmonary and cardiac causes of dyspnea? Then you must suggest more invasive tests or ask for a consult. When you ask for a consult, the examiners will want to know exactly what single question you wish to have answered and what tests you think the consult should include. "A cardiology consult to evaluate cardiac disease" will not suffice. You should say, "I need to know whether the functional status of the heart is contributing to the symptoms of dyspnea." What tests do you suggest? Cath? Pretty invasive. The risk of trauma to the femoral artery and aorta, dye reactions, and expense all argue for something less hazardous as part of the initial workup. MUGA? Not so invasive, and *it answers your question:* the MUGA scan assesses left ventricular function.

The patient presenting for carotid endarterectomy is another catch-22, as he may have cardiac disease. Do you cath him (with its attendant risk), bypass him (with its risk, especially to the brain), then do his carotids? Do you do them both at the same time, then take the blame from the surgeon for the stroke? (You let the pressure get too low on bypass! We should have wakened him after the carotid operation to see how effective the repair was. The heparin helped! The heparin hurt!) Here's a game plan. Go back to basics. Look for a history of angina. If you're stuck, go with a dipyridamole-thallium perfusion scan. That will tell you whether you have myocardium at risk for ischemia. If it is positive, then go to a cardiology consult and let them consider a cath.

Suppose this patient needs a carotid endarterectomy and coronary bypass grafting. What if the examiners press you on which operation you should do first? The examiners like to get you to commit to a position which you cannot defend. Give the pros and cons to each approach and

Preparing for the Anesthesia Orals

say that the final decision can be settled by a discussion with your fellow consultants in neurology, surgery, and cardiology. By then, with any luck, you will hear the knock on the door and your exam will be over.

Incidentally, certain points relevant to carotid endarterectomy patients merit attention. Carotid angiography is performed on patients for a few *specific* indications only: transient ischemic attack (TIA), reversible ischemic neurologic deficit (RIND), or stroke. Don't work up asymptomatic bruits. When discussing an anesthetic plan on patients with carotid stenosis, mention maintaining cerebral perfusion pressure (MAP-CVP) at baseline levels.

How about the femoropopliteal veteran? Your assessment of his exercise tolerance is limited at best, but at least you can rule out clinically severe CHF by seeing if he can lie flat or tolerate a Trendelenburg position. Many peripheral vascular disease patients have diabetes with its consequent risk of silent ischemia. How do you assess the risk of ischemia in such a case?

Assessing risk in the patient prone to silent ischemia is perhaps the toughest question of all. The best we can recommend in this difficult situation is to stick with the freebies: see if the current ECG compared with an old one helps you (it probably won't), then go with a dipyridamole-thallium scan. The problem here is that you'll have to be willing to *do* something about an abnormal result on a dipyridamole-thallium test, like proceed to cath and possible bypass. You may then have stated, in effect, "So before I would let the surgeons do this toe amputation, I would make sure that the patient had a dipyridamole-thallium test. Then if that test were abnormal, I would insist on catheterization and a coronary artery bypass operation."

Common sense tells you that such a course is impractical. It is easy to paint yourself into a corner with the preop evaluation of a patient with possible cardiac disease. A better answer might be, "If the patient were at risk for silent ischemia, but the nature of the operation (minimal fluid shifts, minimal blood loss, short procedure, no expected swings in hemodynamics/sympathetic stimulation) were such that a complete cardiac evaluation were unwarranted, I would gear my anesthetic to minimizing hemodynamic abnormalities that would be detrimental to a patient with coronary disease. In this case of a toe amputation, I would do an ankle block, use a hypobaric spinal with the bad leg up, or else I might use an epidural and dose slowly. I would have pressors and beta-blockers in the room, already drawn up, and would treat hypotension or tachycardia more quickly than I would in other, healthier patients." The examiners may try to dissuade you from your choice. But that *is* the way you treat such patients.

In your everyday practice, you don't go off the deep end on every patient who comes to the OR for a below-knee amputation. Follow your normal practice. Don't try to be extra-invasive in the hope that you will wow the examiners.

11 | AIRWAY, AIRWAY, WHO LOST THE AIRWAY?

You can live without money. You can live without lunch. You can't live without oxygen.

If you learn one lesson in anesthesia, learn your ABCs starting with A for airway. Lose the airway and you've lost the patient. Lose the airway through carelessness on the board exam and you've lost the exam.

How best to prepare? Before you take the exam, think up bad airway scenarios and practice handling them aloud. When you take the exam itself, look over the stem question for tips that the patient may pose a difficult intubation. "Patient required five attempts at intubation by three anesthesiologists." This sort of nuance should make you sit up and take notice.

In case of doubt, do the intubation awake. Of course, certain patients present obstacles to awake intubation (asthmatic, open eye, coronary artery disease), and some patients you just can't intubate awake (a struggling child, the intoxicated patient gritting his teeth and flailing about). Regardless of the obstacles to awake intubation, you must avoid giving relaxants until you are sure you can ventilate. If you lose the airway, if you give a relaxant and then can't ventilate, you may lose the patient. On the boards that may flunk you.

Fiberoptic? Good choice. Why do a "blind" technique when you can see? Even in a patient with coronary disease, you can do a safe fiberoptic intubation. A well-topicalized, well-sedated cardiac patient suffers minimal hemodynamic upset with fiberoptic intubation. Obviously, fiberoptic intubation for every coronary artery bypass graft patient is not routine practice. However, a carefully conducted awake intubation places far less stress on the myocardium than a lost airway and poor ventilation.

Some of the worst dilemmas on the oral boards are bad airway plus something else.

Bad airway plus asthma. Of course you want to avoid instrumenting a lightly anesthetized or nonanesthetized airway in a patient with bronchospastic disease. So how do you tiptoe around it—with a regional? Good choice, but the examiners will find a way to negate any regional technique and force you to confront the difficult airway. This doesn't mean that you should not have regional anesthesia as an appropriate first plan, but you must be ready with a backup plan if you need to convert to a general technique. The patient may refuse a regional technique, blood may appear in the epidural, the spinal may wear off. Some operations under regional aren't really feasible, for example, cholecystectomy. Yes, you can do a high epidural or a spinal for the cholecystectomy, but if the patient has reactive airways disease, he will have a hard time clearing secretions with such a high block.

You can be sure the examiners will create a scenario that goes something like this: The patient gets agitated, you sedate, he gets a big vagal stimulus from a peritoneal stretch, bronchoconstriction worsens. . . . Now the patient is struggling from hypoxia and you have to intubate under the worst of circumstances. Sounds fun, *n'est-ce que pas?*

So what to do with a difficult airway and bronchospastic disease? Certainly do your best to avoid instrumenting the airway. If a regional or mask technique will not suffice (during the oral exam any patient you mask is guaranteed to vomit, aspirate, and require intubation), then take the bull by the horns and tackle a difficult airway head on. Optimize the patient preop and then do the intubation, avoiding the use of muscle relaxants if at all possible. If the stomach isn't full, you can breathe him deep, with a potent inhaled agent and O_2, then take a look. If the intubation is impossible, wake the patient up and start over again. Always leave a way out. Don't sacrifice an unsure airway.

Bad airway and heart disease. You can intubate these patients awake if need be; you just have to have the patient sedated out the wazoo and topicalized well. If during the course of instrumentation bad hemodynamic things happen, treat it as you would at any other time. If tachycardia needs beta-blockade or ST segments need nitroglycerin, then pause for a moment and treat accordingly. Doing an awake intubation does not mean you unlearn all your cardiac skills, you just adapt them to a different setting.

Bad airway, open eye, full stomach. Once again, go with priorities. The airway comes first, but you would hate to see that patient cough and spill vitreous humor. Our solution (and many may disagree) is, spray the patient up, topicalize the upper airway, and *just take a look* with the patient awake. If it looks as though you can intubate, then preoxygenate, give pentothal, succinylcholine (yes, we would), then intubate. If intubation is unsuccessful, the patient will be awake in 5 minutes and you have not lost anything. "Sux?" you say. Although there is a transient increase in extraocular muscle tone, eye contents are not lost. This is preferable to giving, say, vecuronium and instrumenting before the patient is adequately relaxed and having him cough, or mask ventilating a difficult airway for 45 minutes. This whole problem of open eye, full stomach is so popular in the literature that your canal of Schlemm spins. Wrestle with the open eye dilemma yourself and practice it aloud. Have your colleagues pick you apart on it. Defend your plan with practice examiners and you will be able to defend it with real examiners.

Bad airway plus increased intracranial pressure plus full stomach. A bad apple. First, optimize the intracranial pressure (mannitol, Lasix, Decadron), then do your best to secure the airway. Keep in mind that increasing ICP during an awake intubation may kill the patient, losing the airway *surely* will. Both hypoxia and hypercapnia increase ICP dramatically.

The airway is everything. Lose it with nonchalance and you win a return trip to Boardland.

12 | TRAUMALAND

Trauma, man's inhumanity to man, often ends up in the refrigerated surgical suite. If the injury is not too severe, the pathologist doesn't get to interview the patient, you do. When you see a trauma patient on the boards, *don't forget about associated injuries.*

The classic board question involves a kid who fell out of a tree. The planned procedure will be an arm job or computerized axial tomography. Don't miss the boat. Pay attention to your ABCs first, then go over associated injuries from head to toe. A—how is the airway? The kid could have lost consciousness or aspirated, the mouth could be full of blood or teeth. B—breathing. C—circulation and cervical spine. Whenever there is head trauma there may be cervical spine trauma. Make sure you don't pith the patient during intubation. Circulation could be compromised from associated injuries to great vessels, the spleen, or long bones. With head trauma, keep in mind that hypotension almost always has its cause elsewhere, most likely from blood loss in the chest or abdomen.

Once the case has started, hypoxemia may develop. Think aspiration. Anyone with altered consciousness, especially the theoretical patient on the board exam, might have aspirated. The best rapid sequence may still result in aspiration. Several board examinees have met the following sequence on their test: trauma patient, rapid sequence induction without apparent complications, then a clinical sequence consistent with aspiration.

Tension pneumothorax is an ever-present danger in the trauma patient. If the examiners divert your attention on some other point, you may forget to get a chest x-ray. The examiners then jump to the induction sequence. You intubate, place the patient on positive pressure ventilation, and *wham!*—no blood pressure. You Trendelenburg it, ephedrinate the patient, hand ventilate, hang epi, pray to Allah, and—since it's the exam—sacrifice your first-born child. No good. If you do not keep the possibility of tension pneumothorax *in* your head, your examiners will chop *off* your head.

Trauma patients mean associated injuries.

13 | WATERSPORTS

The dumbest kidney is smarter than the brightest nephrologist. If you never get oliguric, you never get anuric.

Wisdom like this is tossed around the OR every day. It underscores the importance of keeping the kidneys humming. You will be asked on your exam to evaluate a patient with low urine output.

Be sure to mention prerenal, renal, and postrenal causes of oliguria. These are listed in Table 2. Know how to differentiate the three entities. Don't give dopamine when the Foley line is kinked, for example. If you've determined that the cause is renal, and is not due to a postrenal obstruction or inadequate prerenal volume or cardiac output, then establish some urine output. You're better off with nonoliguric than oliguric renal failure. Giving renal-dose dopamine is hard to criticize and is a better therapeutic first step than going straight to furosemide. Figure 3 is a flow chart for managing an oliguric patient.

The crux of dialysis questions is to make sure your patient is dialyzed within 24 hours of an elective procedure and has a set of postdialysis labs that include a potassium of less than 5.5 mEq/L. Not only does dialysis get

TABLE 2. *Causes of Postoperative Oliguria*

Prerenal (decreased renal blood flow)
    Hypovolemia
    Decreased renal blood flow due to low cardiac output

Renal (acute tubular necrosis)
    Renal ischemia due to prerenal causes
    Nephrotoxic drugs
    Release of hemoglobin or myoglobin

Postrenal
    Bilateral ureteral obstruction
    Extravasation due to rupture of bladder
    Mechanical (Foley kinked or clotted)

Source: Stoelting RK, Dierdorf SF, McCammon RL. Anesthesia and co-existing disease. New York: Churchill Livingstone, 1988: 433.

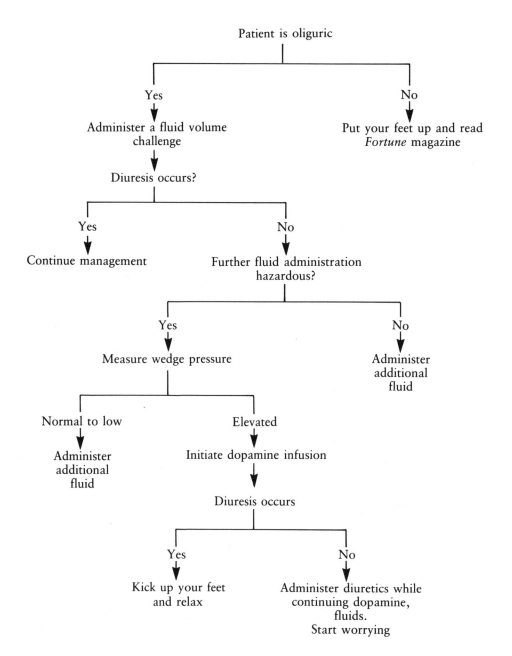

Figure 3
Managing an oliguric patient. (Source: Adapted from Stoelting RK, Dierdorf SF, Mc-Cammon RL. Anesthesia and co-existing disease. New York: Churchill Livingstone, 1988:433.)

rid of all those electrolyte and uremic poisons, it also reverses platelet dysfunction. That platelet dysfunction is worth keeping in mind when you plan a regional technique. The bleeding time is your essential test in that instance.

Know kidney questions. Every examination has them.

Preparing for the Anesthesia Orals

14 | I DON'T KNOW NUTHIN' 'BOUT BIRTHIN' NO BABIES, MIZ SCARLETT

You'd better know a thing or two about epidurals. Obstetrics is a perennial favorite. If you don't see OB in the stem questions, you are sure to see it on the grab-bag part of the test.

Examiners love to hear about normal physiology. ASA refresher courses every year have a "normal physiology of pregnancy" section. What are the physiologic changes of pregnancy?

1. Cardiovascular
   A. Increased intravascular fluid volume
   B. Increased cardiac output
   C. Combination of A and B can lead to cardiac failure in patients with preexisting cardiac disease (especially mitral valve disease)
   D. Increased red blood cell mass (expands less than fluid volume, so hematocrit drops)
   E. Supine hypotension syndrome—the gravid uterus mechanically compresses the aorta and inferior vena cava (remember left uterine displacement)
2. Pulmonary
   A. Increased minute ventilation and oxygen consumption
   B. Decreased FRC and residual volume
   C. Combination of A and B leads to rapid desaturation with loss of airway
3. Gastrointestinal
   A. Decreased gastric emptying
   B. Increased gastric volume
   C. Increased gastric pressure

D. Decreased competence of gastroesophageal junction

E. All of the above—whoops, wrong board exam

F. A, B, C, and D mean the stomach is always considered full after the first trimester

4. Neurologic

A. Increased engorgement of epidural vessels

B. Decreased local anesthetic dosing needed for intrathecal and epidural anesthesia

C. A and B increase the likelihood of intravascular injection or high spinal in the pregnant patient

Although many other physiologic changes are associated with pregnancy, the changes just listed are the most important. The examiners will ask you about them.

Pre-eclampsia has pathology from head to toe:

A. Head—intracranial bleeding, visual changes, headaches

B. Airway—increased venous engorgement and glottic edema resulting in a decreased glottic opening

C. Heart and lungs—leaky capillaries, pulmonary edema, possible LV dysfunction

D. Liver—potential rupture of Glisson's capsule

E. Kidneys—oliguria, proteinuria, or renal failure may result from systemic vasoconstriction and hypovolemia

F. Blood—coagulopathy (especially thrombocytopenia)

Given these changes in pre-eclampsia, match procedure to pathology. Regional techniques require a recent platelet count and adequate volume replacement with adequate monitoring. The exam tends to concentrate on your choice of and rationale for monitoring. "When will you use an arterial line and/or a pulmonary artery catheter?" is a common query. In mild pre-eclampsia, routine monitoring, careful hydration and titration of local anesthetic is sufficient. However, with oliguria a CVP line is essential. With severe pre-eclampsia, an arterial line is indicated due to blood pressure lability and the need to maintain uteroplacental perfusion (minimum BP of 140/90 mm Hg) and to quickly treat hypertension that could lead to cerebral hemorrhage. If there is evidence of cardiopulmonary dysfunction (impaired oxygenation, oliguria, dyspnea, or rales) or continued oliguria in the presence of a normal CVP, the possibility of LV dysfunction or nonagreement of the CVP with the PAOP mandates the use of a pulmonary artery catheter.

Given the coagulopathy, you must check coagulation parameters (prothrombin time, partial thromboplastin time, platelets) to avoid the risk of an epidural hematoma in pre-eclamptic patients.

Failed intubation is the ultimate toughie in OB. Failed intubation without fetal distress is no biggie: wake the patient up and then try awake intubation. Failed intubation with fetal distress is a dilemma with *no good, clear-cut, "right" answer*. All *we* can do is list the pros and cons of the various options. All *you* can do is pick one and stick with it. This is the classic example of a board question with no absolutely correct response.

1. Wake the patient up and intubate her awake at your leisure. The thinking here is: the mother is your patient, do what's safest for your patient. The baby, of course, can be in ongoing distress during this time.

2. Mask the patient all the way through with cricoid pressure. This runs the risk of the patient aspirating, but many C-sections have been done by mask technique without aspiration. The mask technique also runs the risk of having to intubate later if airway obstruction develops.

3. Do a tracheostomy or a cricothyrotomy right away. This carries all the risks of emergently slashing a throat, does not ensure that you will get the airway (since a tracheostomy is not always *successful*), but it *is* a last resort if you're in a jam.

4. Wake the patient up and do the C-section under local infiltration with ketamine sedation. *Ouch!* This could be a disaster, with the patient thrashing around in agony, possibly vomiting, and the surgeons struggling with a rollicking operative field.

5. Wake the patient up and do a spinal. The patient might not be able to tolerate it (say she has a bleeding previa or abruption) and a spinal burns up time. If the mother is hemodynamically stable and the spinal is done swiftly and successfully with the level not going too high, then it does get you out of a jam.

Do *you* want to pick any of those options? Obviously not—no one does. You must, however, be ready to answer this most difficult of questions. We have not provided an exhaustive list of possible answers. You might discuss with your colleagues this scenario of a failed intubation with fetal distress—they may have a better response than those we've listed.

For OB, know the normal physiology, the anesthetic considerations for pre-eclampsia, and your response to a failed intubation.

I Don't Know Nuthin' 'bout Birthin' No Babies, Miz Scarlett

15 | LITTLE RASCALS

Kids get blue real quick.

Kids don't take Swans.

Kids don't listen when you say, "Just a little pressure now."

Kids do the darndest things.

Examiners are likely to pin you down on the following pediatric questions:

- Bleeding tonsil
- Epiglottitis
- Neonatal resuscitation
- Normal vital signs and lab values in children
- Malignant hyperthermia

The bleeding tonsil is the quintessential kiddie question. The trap the examiners lay for you goes like this: The patient is upset, bleeding, and needs emergency re-exploration to stop the bleeding, and the IV line is infiltrated. The foolish person says, "Well, if I upset him too much he'll cry and make the bleeding worse, so I'll just mask him *a little bit.*" That will tend to kill the patient *a little bit.* Bleeding-tonsil patients have all bled an unknown amount and have swallowed the blood; thus they are hypovolemic and have a full stomach. Don't be duped by this classic trap. Do whatever is necessary for an IV (cutdown, central line, surgeons pitching in). Replace the volume. Do your induction with a full stomach in mind (awake intubation or rapid sequence). Most practitioners would prefer a rapid sequence induction with ketamine over an awake intubation. An awake intubation in a struggling child is likely to stir up more bleeding and obliterate your visualization.

Epiglottitis usually appears on the exam in the form of a trap: "But the ENT man really wants to take an indirect look in the ER." Instrumenting the airway in a child with epiglottitis invites catastrophic airway closure. If epiglottitis is suspected, the patient must be examined in the OR, with the ENT surgeon ready to do a tracheostomy. Then the patient must be breathed down and examined only after adequate anesthetic depth has been established. Don't be duped into examining the child outside of the OR.

Oxygen, oxygen, oxygen, and respiratory support are the key points of neonatal resuscitation. Bicarbonate is evil in neonates (hypotension, hyperosmolality, intraventricular hemorrhage). Apgar scores (less than 3 means intubation, 4–6 means mask support) appear on exams. If you can't place an IV line in a neonate, you can give epinephrine, lidocaine, and atropine via the endotracheal tube. Drugs and cardioversion all take a back seat to adequate ventilatory support in neonatal resuscitation. Essentially any arrest in this age group is respiratory in origin.

Memorize normal vital signs at various ages (Table 3)—you look like a real geek when you smugly say, "Looks a little tachy to me" and you can't even say what a normal heart rate is. No one can memorize all those values cold, but a fair knowledge of them will get you by. If you don't anesthetize children routinely, look over that table again. You don't want to get caught short on a question pertaining to vital signs.

Another question you may field is, "How do you assess the volume status of a child?" Placing central lines in children is not easy; therefore you must have a way of clinically assessing volume depletion. Table 4 gives the clues.

Pediatric emergencies are a favorite for the grab-bag session of the oral exam.

TABLE 3. *Normal Values for Vital Signs in Pediatric Patients*

Age	Average (range)
Normal heart rate (bpm)	
Newborn	120 (100–170)
1–12 months	120 (80–160)
2 years	110 (80–130)
4 years	100 (80–120)
6 years	100 (75–115)
Normal blood pressure (mm Hg)	
Newborn:	
Premature	44/24
Full term	49/26
3–10 days	75 systolic
6 months	95 systolic
4 years	98/57
6 years	110/60

Source: Steward DJ. Manual of pediatric anesthesia, 2d edition. New York: Churchill Livingstone, 1985: 21.

Preparing for the Anesthesia Orals

TABLE 4. *Signs of Volume Depletion in Pediatric Patients*

	Degree of Dehydration (in % of body weight)		
	5%	10%	15%
Skin turgor	−	− −	− − −
Sunken fontanelle	−	− −	− − −
Skin color	Pale	Gray	Mottled
Mucous membranes	Dry	Very dry	Parched
Urine	−	− −	Anuric
Heart rate	Normal	↑	↑ ↑

Source: Gregory GA. Pediatric anesthesia. In Miller RD (ed), Anesthesia, 2d edition. New York: Churchill Livingstone, 1986: 1771.

Pyloric stenosis is a medical management problem, never a surgical emergency. The patient has a full stomach. Correction of the hypovolemic, hypochloremic, hypokalemic metabolic alkalosis must precede any surgical procedure. Suck out the stomach before you induce. Realize that suctioning never guarantees an empty stomach, then proceed with a rapid sequence induction. Awake intubation is also an option, but most of these children struggle too much with an awake intubation.

Congenital diaphragmatic hernia gives any nonpediatric anesthesiologist shortness of breath. This is a surgical emergency, and you can't wriggle out of doing the case even if you say, "I'll call Joe, who usually does kids in my group practice." Joe will be the first anesthesiologist on the space shuttle and you'll be the only person on earth who can save the kid. For monitoring, have a right-sided A-line and pulse oximeter to follow the oxygen saturation of the blood supplying the brain and the eyes. Blood from the persistent fetal circulation contributes arterial blood to the left side, and you want to know what's happening on the right side, the side that reflects brain oxygenation and the development of retrolental fibroplasia.

The child with congenital diaphragmatic hernia will present with a scaphoid abdomen and abdominal gas appearing in the left thorax. That gas must be sucked out by nasogastric tube as soon as possible. Positive pressure by mask may further fill those abdominal contents with gas and make ventilation difficult. An awake intubation with gentle positive pressure (<25 cm H_2O) is the wisest course. The most important consideration in congenital diaphragmatic hernia is: don't try to expand the hypoplastic lung. That may result in a pneumothorax on the side of the good lung. *Pneumothorax, pneumothorax, and pneumothorax* are the first three possibilities to consider when things go kablooey pre-, intra-, or postop. These children are most susceptible to dropping a lung and developing hypoxemia.

Patients with congenital diaphragmatic hernia can also develop hypoxemia from *shunting blood away from* the lungs. If pulmonary artery vascular resistance is increased, then blood can shunt away from the lungs through a patent ductus arteriosus (PDA). Pulmonary artery resistance is increased by hypoxia, hypercapnia, crying, acidosis, cold, and light anesthesia. The increased pulmonary tone will exacerbate persistent fetal circulation through the PDA and worsen hypoxemia. Thus, hypoxemia can occur by several mechanisms. Treatment consists of optimizing factors that increase pulmonary tone. Keep the patient warm, quickly treat suspected pneumothorax, keep the patient anesthetized (these fragile patients may not tolerate inhaled agents), and keep the metabolic milieu normal.

Malignant hyperthermia (MH) appears in one of two ways on the exam. The first scenario entails a patient undergoing elective surgery who has a family member with a history of, or highly suggestive of, malignant hyperthermia. The second scenario entails an elective procedure on a patient with a vague and undefined history of intraoperative or postoperative fever, the extent of which can rarely be determined. The questions you will be asked will center on preoperative testing: Will you really send him to Philadelphia? Will you test the entire family? Will you do a nontriggering anesthetic without testing? Will you give prophylactic dantrolene? How about masseter spasm?

The following answers are based on a conversation with the Malignant Hyperthermia Hotline. After reading ad nauseum about these controversial questions and receiving widely conflicting answers from scores of our colleagues, we telephoned the source.

Preop dantrolene   Don't give dantrolene preop. Have it available and give it early if signs develop.

Exotic trips to faraway places for biopsies   If you suspect MH, send the patient for a biopsy only for nonmedical reasons (can't get life insurance, a pilot's license, an appointment to the armed services). Also, send the patient for a biopsy if the local doctors refuse to treat him. You as a consultant anesthesiologist know that the biopsy itself carries risk and expense. You as a consultant know that the biopsy is imperfect, and that even if it reads negative it may be a false negative. But if the patient's medical treatment back home is such that no anesthesiologist there will anesthetize him without a biopsy, then send the patient for a biopsy. You yourself will still give a *nontriggering anesthetic* even if the biopsy is negative.

Testing the family   Test the family only for the nonmedical reasons listed above.

Masseter spasm   Masseter spasm must be considered a pre-MH sign. Stop the surgery unless life, limb, or sight will be destroyed. If they are threatened, proceed with a nontriggering anesthetic and maintain a high index of suspicion for the first hint of MH. Even though patients with masseter spasm are difficult to intubate, you should be able to ventilate. Future anesthetics for such patients will be nontriggering, unless you have a fondness for the judicial system.

What is safe?   Essentially anything except for succinylcholine and potent inhaled agents.

Treatment   Stop the anesthetic, get a clean machine, give 100% O_2, give dantrolene, hyperventilate, correct the metabolic abnormalities, monitor and treat urine output. The signs of MH are essentially the signs of a metabolic supernova: tachycardia (earliest sign), hyperpnea and increased CO_2 production, oxygen desaturation, mottled skin, increased temperature (late sign). Attempts at spontaneous ventilation by a supposedly paralyzed patient are a common hint on the exam.

In summary, the Big Kahunas in pediatric anesthesia are MH, bleeding tonsils, normal vital signs, volume depletion, and congenital diaphragmatic hernia.

Now beat it kid, you bother me.

16 | ROCKIN' ROUND THE BLOCK

When the clock strikes one we're gonna have some fun, we're gonna treat toxicity when the clock strikes one.

Careful as you are on the exam, your local anesthetic will go toxic. Aspirate frequently, ask for premonitory symptoms, give a test dose, and you will still get a toxic reaction. Check the cuff when you are doing a Bier block. Be ready to explain how to resuscitate a patient from an overdose of local anesthetics. Slice it, dice it, make it into mounds of julienne fries—whatever regional technique you pick on the oral board can go intravascular.

First things first: give oxygen and support the airway. Often this is all you will have to do. Unconscious? Apneic? Don't panic, you may get by with just masking the airway, you don't necessarily have to intubate. Support the ABCs, consider pentothal or succinylcholine if the seizures are so severe that they interfere with ventilation. Volume and pressors are necessary if blood pressure drops. CPR? If it's needed, it's needed. Don't lose your cool if your case goes all the way to CPR. That doesn't mean you flunked the exam, it just means that now the examiners want to test your knowledge of cardiopulmonary resuscitation. ABC, ABC, ABC.

Worried about doses of local anesthetics? Believe it or not, the examiners can't actually press you too hard on doses. In the real world you can look these up, and you *do*. They won't nail you if you can't remember how many cc's to give. Also, most anesthetics are packaged so that 1 cc of brand X is equivalent to drug Y used for the same purpose. If you do make a reference to looking things up, know where you plan to look. "Since I have not done an axillary block in some time, I would look in the Mass. General handbook for how many cc's of mepivacaine would be appropriate for this small patient" versus "I don't know, I'd look it up somewhere."

Know the differences and advantages of the various regional techniques: interscalene, axillary, and Bier blocks for the upper extremity, spinal and epidural for the nether regions.

How about those upper extremity blocks? You don't have to write a thesis, just the normal facts that differentiate them. Interscalene is best for procedures at or above the elbow, axillary is best for procedures below the elbow, and a Bier block has the advantage of almost always ending up in the right place. Was that so hard? Interscalenes have the disadvantage of any neck stick: pneumothorax, carotid puncture, intrathecal tracking. Axillary blocks often puncture the axillary artery, which may continue to bleed. Bier blocks are limited by the patient's tolerance of tourniquet pain. If the tourniquet should malfunction on a Bier block, the patient gets a large intravenous dose of local anesthetic.

Epidural versus spinal? Epidural often provides inadequate perineal anesthesia such as that required for a urologic procedure and inadequate ankle anesthesia (L5–S1). The ability to redose and slowly build up a block is a real plus for epidurals. The controllability inherent in a slowly set up block helps the patient who can't handle fast volume shifts. Epidurals have the disadvantage of using larger doses of local anesthetics. If those higher doses are injected intrathecally, a total spinal results; large doses mistakenly given intravascularly yield cardiovascular collapse.

Spinal techniques have the advantage of lower doses, thus less possibility of overdose. The dense block provides good perineal analgesia, but the rapid sympathetic block may hurt a patient with poor compensatory mechanisms (myocardial dysfunction, aortic stenosis, hypovolemia). Postspinal headaches, seen most often in young patients, are another drawback.

Preparing for the Anesthesia Orals

17 | THE EYES HAVE IT

Disaster lurks in the eye room. Keep your guard up. Be ready to handle the ultimate disaster: the patient who suddenly can't lie flat anymore and is coughing after the surgeons have already opened the eye.

Sedating this patient runs a grave risk. He could be agitated from hypoxemia or congestive heart failure, so further sedation could lead to worse agitation. If you are struggling with an open eye patient, induce general anesthesia. Control that airway, don't try to tiptoe around it. Yes, the ophthalmologist *can* drape the open eye well enough for you to intubate the patient without injuring the eye.

The other generic eye question is the oculocardiac reflex. The afferent pathway is trigeminal and the efferent is vagal. The oculocardiac reflex does exhibit tachyphylaxis, so once you tell the surgeons to release pressure on the globe or extraocular muscle, the bradycardia may disappear and reapplication of pressure on the globe may not give such a dramatic bradycardia the second time. If, however, the bradycardia persists, *once you have ensured adequacy of ventilation,* then atropine is appropriate.

18 | PÂTÉ

The slightly elevated SGOT is vexing. Do you cancel for a teeny elevation in the SGOT, or do you forge ahead and risk hepatic necrosis? What rattles you about an elevated SGOT is the fear that the patient may have an active inflammatory process in the liver. Proceeding in the face of ongoing liver damage may worsen liver function. You must know if the inflammation has peaked and is now decreasing.

Repeat the SGOT before you proceed with an elective case. If the SGOT is decreasing, then the liver inflammation should also be decreasing and you can proceed with surgery. If the test shows continuing or increasing liver damage, then defer elective surgery until the inflammation subsides. A GI consult is the way to determine when best to proceed in such a case. The question on the top of the consult sheet may read, "This man has had an SGOT in the 200 range for 2 weeks straight. We want to minimize any hepatic insult. When is the best time to proceed with surgery?"

What other tests do you need in the patient with liver disease? Pursue those liver functions with an impact on anesthesia:

1. Glucose hemostasis is off-kilter, so you have to make sure to follow the glucose level intraop.
2. Albumin production drops, with all the attendant pharmacoavailability concerns, so check the albumin.
3. Coagulation parameters may be markedly decreased. Check a prothrombin time.
4. Ammonia levels? They can be elevated in the last stages of terminal liver disease, but no one would take you to task on an ammonia level.
5. Blood gases? Sure as shooting. Cirrhotic patients can have pulmonary shunts with resultant large alveolar-arterial gradients.
6. Sodium? All cirrhotics have increased total body water, with total body sodium up and sodium concentration down. The increased body water also alters the volume of distribution of drugs. Neuromuscular agents must be delivered at higher initial doses to overcome this "diluting" factor.

Which anesthetic agent or technique best protects the liver? How do you respond when the GI specialist says, "OK for surgery but *just* use a spinal"? All anesthetics decrease liver blood flow and can exacerbate pre-existing hepatic insufficiency, so *just* a spinal is really no safer than a general anesthetic. More important than the anesthetic, actually, is the proximity of the surgical site to the liver. Liver blood flow drops more than with a cholecystectomy than with a hernia. The best way to describe your anesthetic plan is, "Once the patient is deemed at the least possible risk for operation, I would conduct a (general, epidural, or spinal) anesthetic, paying most attention to maintaining high oxygenation and optimal fluid status. The actual choice of which technique I use is less important than the support I give during the operation." Bite your tongue, but you are saying in effect, "I would avoid hypotension and hypoxia."

Which anesthetic agent will you choose? Lurking in that question somewhere is the halothane hepatitis issue.

1. Incidence—1/35,000. Not seen in children.
2. Most susceptible—overweight females with previous recent exposure to a halothane anesthetic.
3. Worse in cirrhotics?—no.
4. Always to blame?—no, a thorough search often turns up another cause, such as cytomegalovirus, surgical compression of the liver, or blood transfusion.

One liver question is a giveaway. Where are local anesthetics metabolized? Esters in the plasma, amides in the liver.

19 | COLLOID IS THICKER THAN WATER

When do you transfuse?

"Dr. Smith, the child has a hematocrit of 25. Would you transfuse?" The wise Dr. Smith considers the patient's underlying illnesses, the rate of blood loss, the extent of the procedure, and says no, confident in his view on transfusion. "How about 23?" Dr. Smith starts to pale. "Well, um, that's getting down there [ulp], but still no." "21?" "Now that's getting pretty low, yes, I would transfuse at exactly 21, but not 22!"

Sooner or later, you must pick a cutoff point for transfusion. Adherence to a fixed hematocrit is applicable only for an individual patient. You can't generalize. For instance, if the patient has cardiopulmonary dysfunction that will impair oxygen delivery, then a hematocrit of at least 30 is a reasonable cutoff. If a healthy 20-year-old has trauma and associated anemia, we would not give blood until the hematocrit fell to 22. This is in accord with current NIH consensus recommendations. Stand firm with a preset number only after you give careful consideration to all the other factors associated with oxygen supply and demand: cardiac output, sepsis, overall health of the patient, age, anticipated blood loss.

> "Just hang it, I said," barks the burly orthopod to the diminutive aerobics instructor-turned-anesthesiologist. "I'm telling you, this guy needs fresh frozen!"

This scene, played over and over again in ORs from Nantucket to Tallahassee, may appear on your test. Stand your ground on the exam. Patients with proven coagulopathies need fresh frozen. Hanging fresh frozen plasma after a certain number of units of blood is not scientific, nor is it effective. After all, the most common cause of bleeding in cases of large transfusions is a dilutional thrombocytopenia. Transfusing fresh frozen without proving a need is knee-jerk medicine, not thinking medicine, and certainly not the response of a consultant anesthesiologist.

One last question on fluids is colloid versus crystalloid. Choose whichever you want (crystalloid is cheaper), but know that there are no good outcome studies to recommend one over the other.

Preparing for the Anesthesia Orals

20 | SYDNEY GREENSTREET PLAYS THE FAT MAN

Obesity is an exam favorite. Examiners often get heavy-handed with this big topic.

Organize your thoughts on obesity by going from head-to-toe.

1. *Head/Psychiatric.* The obese patient, more than 50% above ideal body weight, may have a passive-aggressive behavior pattern. Preoperative line placement may be extra difficult if the patient refuses to cooperate.

2. *Airway.* Assess the oral/pharyngeal/neck anatomy. Extra soft tissue may prohibit adequate extension of the neck. A thick neck may obscure a receding chin. Large breasts may inhibit the ability to manipulate the handle of the laryngoscope. Pharyngeal obstruction may occur with induction, and the heavy chest may make mask ventilation impossible. Mask ventilation is best avoided anyway because obese patients are at high risk for having a full stomach.

   Awake intubation is an acceptable answer to the problem of intubating the morbidly obese in almost all circumstances. If the induction must be done prior to instrumenting the airway (because of increased intracranial pressure or a bad heart, for instance), then you must be prepared for a failed intubation and inability to ventilate. Have plan B formulated: an ENT surgeon nearby, ready to perform an immediate tracheostomy in case you can't intubate or ventilate. It's easier to call across the room than across town for the ENT surgeon.

3. *Lungs.* The combination of decreased functional residual capacity (FRC) and large oxygen demand results in quick desaturation following loss of the airway. A classic mistake on the exam is to say, "Once monitors were placed, I would do a rapid sequence induction using cricoid pressure." "Oh, a rapid sequence?" "Yes, I'm concerned about a full stomach, since any patient of this size should be regarded as having

a full stomach." The examiner responds, "The patient desaturates, you can't intubate, ventricular fibrillation occurs, and the patient dies. You forgot to preoxygenate, DOCTOR!"

Pulmonary function tests show a restrictive pattern. A baseline blood gas is necessary in the preop evaluation, since the patient may be pickwickian (sleep apnea, chronic hypoventilation). The presence of chronic hypoxemia, possible CO_2 retention, and decreased FRC all lead to increased pulmonary vascular resistance.

4. *Heart.* Longstanding pulmonary hypertension from hyoxemia can lead to cor pulmonale. The clue that appears in the stem question is the hematocrit. On the oral exam, an obese patient often will have an elevated hematocrit, clueing you to hunt for chronic hypoxemia and its sequelae. Obese patients have an increased incidence of hypertension and associated left ventricular dysfunction. Biventricular failure, if present, would mandate invasive monitoring with evaluation of preload, contractility, and afterload of each ventricle.

5. *Gastrointestinal.* The large pannus causes increased abdominal pressure which, combined with increased gastric volume, makes the obese prone to acid aspiration. Wisdom dictates pretreatment with metoclopramide and ranitidine (night before and morning of surgery).

Expect questions on the obese patient. It's not over 'til the fat lady sings.

21 | SAMPLE QUESTIONS

OK, you're a big kid now, armed with an approach to a lot of hard questions. Time to graduate and use your knowledge. The best way to practice answering is to practice answering. What follows is a list of questions patterned after the board questions. Any similarity to actual questions is coincidental.

We will go through the sequence which might follow such a question. There are two ways to approach the dissection of a stem question:

1. *Word/phrase approach.* Take each word/phrase in the stem and anticipate why that item has been included and what questions will be asked pertaining to that word or phrase. This technique follows the order in which the information is given.
2. *Preop/intraop/postop approach.* Map out the preop, intraop, and postop problems you anticipate with the patient. This technique follows the order in which the exam will be given.

Using only a general knowledge of anesthesia and our familiarity with the oral board mode of questioning, we have constructed a comprehensive review of the most likely points to be touched on during an oral exam. The majority of what we have written should be familiar to you.

Use the blank pages. Practice writing your own answers.

Our answers alternate between a word/phrase analysis and a preop/intraop/postop approach. Your answers may be different. They may be better. In any case, be able to defend what you say.

CASE 1 *(word/phrase approach)*

An 85-year-old, 68 kg male sustains minor head trauma after falling from a swingset. He has a transient syncopal episode after the fall. Three days later he presents in the ER with a history of vomiting and confusion. An emergency craniotomy is scheduled. BP 170/90; HR 48; T 38°C; BUN 55.

85 years old   All the considerations for geriatric patients: increased sensitivity (pharmacokinetic rather than actually pharmacodynamic) to pentothal, decreased clearance of all drugs, decreased reserve in all organ systems.

68 kg   Normal body weight.

minor head trauma   Not minor if he's got all those signs of increased intracranial pressure (ICP). Think associated injuries, especially of the cervical spine.

transient syncopal episode   Must have been quite a knock. Again, cervical spine injury should cross your mind. Start thinking about increased ICP.

vomiting and confusion   *Really* start thinking about increased ICP. The vomiting reminds you that patients with increased ICP after trauma should be considered to have a full stomach.

emergency craniotomy   They will ask you about how to monitor the brain (intracranial bolt monitoring of ICP is especially efficacious in head trauma), how to protect the brain (furosemide, mannitol; no dexamethasone or glucose solutions with trauma-induced increases in ICP), how to diagnose venous air embolism (in order of sensitivity: transesophageal echo, Doppler over the precordium, end-tidal nitrogen, end-tidal CO_2 and arterial to end-tidal CO_2 gradient, increased pulmonary artery pressures, ECG pattern of right heart strain, hemodynamic collapse).

What to do if an air embolus occurs? (Memorize this and you'll score big points. You almost can't fail if you slam-dunk the question on venous air embolism.) Supportive measures. 100% oxygen while flooding the field, call for help, and aspirate through your multiorifice CVP line. Raise CVP by fluid loading, no PEEP or you might raise CVP at the risk of sending a paradoxical air embolus through a probe-patent foramen ovale, get ready for cardiopulmonary resuscitation. Have epinephrine ready and try to position the patient for CPR.

Know how to handle positioning, especially sitting: slow assumption of position to prevent hemodynamic collapse secondary to lower-extremity sequestration of intravascular volume. Baroreceptor reflexes are ablated under anesthesia.

BP 170/90, P 48   You will certainly be asked whether you want to decrease the blood pressure. Don't be fooled, the blood pressure is up for a reason: the patient has increased ICP with a reflex bradycardia. If you lower the blood pressure you will *decrease the cerebral perfusion pressure* (examiners love to hear that). Cerebral perfusion pressure = mean arterial pressure − intracranial pressure.

T 38   Vital signs are vital, they are all given to you for a reason. The patient's temperature is elevated, increasing his cerebral metabolic rate. Cool the patient—Tylenol, don't warm the IV fluids—to decrease the cerebral metabolic rate of oxygen consumption ($CMRO_2$). Also, the temperature may be elevated from an infection, such as pneumonia secondary to aspiration during the loss of consciousness. Check the chest x-ray.

BUN 55   You won't get lots of lab data on the stem question, but the examiners will ask you about the lab data you do get. Why the high BUN? Dehydration from vomiting, preexisting renal disease, or reabsorption of a hematoma are all possible. Is this a new abnormality? Try to get old lab values as a baseline.

How should you actually answer the question, "Why the high BUN?" Don't waste time pecking around for more information, get on with the answer. Control the exam and say, "I would try to get old labs as a baseline. Assuming that this is a new abnormality, my most likely diagnosis would be dehydration secondary to vomiting. I would then look to see if further lab tests—such as an arterial blood gas, potassium chloride, and creatinine—confirmed that diagnosis." The examiners will then ask you what those further lab tests would show. You say, "Hypochloremic, hypokalemic metabolic alkalosis with a BUN/creatinine ratio >20/1."

This method of answering is the most efficient. Create your own differential and then answer it. Don't get in a tug of war with the examiners, such as:

"Why the high BUN?"

"Well, does the patient have old labs?"

"Yes."

"Does he have a blood gas?"

"Yes, it shows alkalosis."

"Metabolic, or what?"

"Metabolic."

"It could be from vomiting. Does he have a bump on his head?"

"Yes."

"Well it could be from that."

This method is slow and tortuous. You don't really cut to the heart of the matter and convince the examiners that you have a grip on the topic.

There you have a word/phrase analysis of a stem question. Each scrap of the stem question gives rise to important points and difficult questions. Though short, the stem is packed with information.

CASE 2 *(preop/intraop/postop approach)*

A 59-year-old, 53 kg female has been hospitalized for 2 weeks with small bowel obstruction and is scheduled for laparotomy. Hyperalimentation solution is being delivered via a subclavian catheter. She has a long smoking history. BP 130/70; HR 75; T 37.5°C rectal.

PREOP

    1. Labs The weight of 53 kg may indicate malnourishment and dehydration, therefore check albumin, electrolytes, glucose, and urine output. Since she has been in the hospital for 2 weeks, she must be colonized by every resistant gram-negative germ on earth, so check for signs or lab data of infection. Hyperalimentation can cause liver abnormalities, so check SGOT and alkaline phosphatase. A room air blood gas is useful, and PFTs would be indicated if the patient were symptomatic (wheezing, history of dyspnea, or chronic cough with purulent sputum production) as a result of her smoking history.

2. Consults No other specialists need be consulted.

3. Further medical treatment Keep the nasogastric tube (NG) decompressing the gut. Assess fluid status and volume resuscitate.

INTRAOP

1. Special considerations Given her state of malnutrition, there will be high availability of protein-bound drugs.

The patient is likely to be dehydrated from third spacing and NG suction.

2. Monitors You don't have to list your routine monitoring methods unless the examiners specifically ask for them. Standard of care is BP, ECG, temperature, pulse oximeter, breath sounds, FIO_2, and an anesthesiologist/anesthetist present at all times in the OR.

A capnogram is not yet considered a routine monitoring aid but is always useful, especially in a rapid sequence where intubation of the esophagus could lead to aspiration.

A Foley catheter should be placed to monitor urine output as an indirect assessment of volume status.

A CVP is debatable. If the urine output has been inadequate and a preop fluid challenge does not increase it, only then is a CVP necessary.

3. Induction Suction the NG, then pull it. (Some argue to keep the NG after suctioning; both answers are acceptable.) In any event, the integrity of the gastroesophageal junction is compromised. Check the fluid status to make sure you do not induce anesthesia in a hypovolemic patient. Use rapid sequence induction if the airway is normal, awake intubation if the airway is abnormal.

4. Maintenance Enflurane/oxygen, supplemented by narcotics. The examiners will ask you why you choose a particular agent. In this case, the patient is at risk for liver abnormalities from hyperalimentation and an abdominal operation. Therefore avoid halothane to avoid confusing the differential diagnosis of postoperative liver dysfunction. Isoflurane is acceptable but more expensive. Avoid nitrous oxide, which will diffuse into air trapped in the bowel and increase bowel distention.

Think before you speak. In this case, don't mention halothane hepatitis unless you are prepared to discuss it.

5. Emergence Since the patient has a full stomach, she must be fully awake before extubation.

6. Intraop problems

a. *Failed intubation* (always be prepared for this). Keep cricoid pressure, ventilate by mask, let the patient awaken, then perform an awake intubation.

b. *Hypotension.* Ensure adequacy of ventilation, turn on 100% oxygen, turn off all anesthetic agents, check the ECG. Then give fluids, place patient in Trendelenburg position (controversial), give ephedrine.

c. *Aspiration* (even a perfectly acceptable anesthetic technique can result in an adverse event during your exam). Suction with the head to the side, intubate, suction the trachea, check the pH of the aspirate. Bronchoscopy is indicated only if you cannot ventilate. No steroids, no antibiotics. Institute supportive therapy intraoperatively. This includes placement of an arterial line for frequent blood gas monitoring and administration of PEEP if necessary.

POSTOP

1. Pain Patient-controlled analgesia (PCA) would be a good option. Since the patient will not go to an ICU postop, do not use intrathecal or epidural narcotics (late respiratory depression).

Again, think before you speak. If all you know is IV and IM narcotic administration, don't bring up the unfamiliar topics of PCA, intrathecal, or epidural narcotics. If pressed on this or any other unfamiliar topic, say, "I am not familiar with that technique. I would use a technique I *am* familiar with." Don't BS the examiners—they'll see right through you and rip you to shreds.

2. Low urine output Check the Foley and give a fluid challenge. If no urine output results after an aggressive fluid challenge, place a CVP line. If there is no increase in urine after an adequate CVP, then, if there is any indication of cardiac disease, go to a pulmonary artery catheter and make sure filling pressures and cardiac output are OK before giving furosemide.

3. Hypoxemia First check the airway and administer supplemental oxygen. If the patient aspirated intraop, then continue supportive care, guided by frequent blood gases. Postoperative ventilation with PEEP may be necessary. Check the chest x-ray for a lesion consistent with aspiration. Recall that aspiration may not appear on the chest film for up to 18 hours. Also consider other common, treatable causes of hypoxemia: pneumothorax, misplaced endotracheal tube, atelectasis, bronchospasm. PEEP may adversely affect the patient's hemodynamics. Replace volume guided by central monitoring trends; absolute numbers may be elevated with PEEP.

There you have an example of each kind of analysis of the stem question. If you continue to read what we have written, you are guaranteed to learn a small fraction of what we have to say. If you jump into the active mode, however, you are sure to learn more. For the next 18 stem questions, we will leave blanks for you to fill in. *After* you have thought them through for yourself and filled them in, look at our answers. The blank spaces we leave will get progressively longer so you can get more and more involved in the answering process.

Practice writing your thoughts down. On the actual exam, you will have 10 minutes to write down your thoughts on a piece of paper before you step into the room with the examiners.

CASE 3 *(word/phrase approach)*

A 20-year-old, 5′0″ tall, 85 kg female is admitted for elective C-section. The last trimester has been complicated by hypertension and proteinuria. Current Rx includes magnesium sulfate and hydralazine. BP 145/95; HR 85; R 16.

85 kg, 5′0″ tall, and pregnant   Obese. If the patient were not pre-eclamptic, then an ___Awake___ intubation would be safest. In this case, the risk of severe hypertension and intracranial hemorrhage argue against an ___Awake___ intubation. Perform a rapid sequence induction.

    FRC is reduced by both ___pregnancy___ and ___obesity___ _____. Oxygen consumption is up secondary to ___Full term preg___. The time to arterial desaturation after preoxygenation (don't forget preoxygenation!) will be very short indeed. The risk of aspiration is ___increased___ _____ from obesity and pregnancy.

elective C-section   The patient is NPO but the stomach is still ___Full___. Given the ___Aspiration___ risk, administer a nonparticulate antacid. Cimetidine, ranitidine, and metoclopramide have not been reported to cause adverse effects on the fetus; however, long-term effects are ___unknown___. I would not give these drugs. [This is a controversial answer.]

hypertension and proteinuria   Pre-eclampsia, pre-eclampsia, pre-eclampsia! She needs ___IV fluid, recent platelet count___ _____ before an epidural is placed. If she has oliguria unresponsive to fluid administration, she needs a ___CVP cath___. If there are signs of congestive heart failure or decreased oxygenation (possible pulmonary edema), a ___PA cath___ should be placed. She may be difficult to intubate due to upper airway and vocal cord ___Edema___. Renal failure may be associated with this condition. ___Intracranial Hemorrhage___ with severe hypertension can be a fatal complication.

magnesium Can cause a floppy child. The floppiness can be reversed in the newborn with time or with ___Calcium chl.___

BP 145/95 Severe pre-eclampsia (minimum BP 160/110) warrants an arterial line. Unless this patient has other signs of severe pre-eclampsia (___seizures___, ___visual Δ's___, ___+4 proteinuria___, ___severe oliguria___), she does not need an arterial line.

Don't peek yet. Fill in what you think are good answers. Remember, your answers may differ from ours (shown in bold type), and may be better than ours.

~~~~~~~~~~~~~~~~~~~~~~~

85 kg, 5′0″ tall, and pregnant Obese. If the patient were not pre-eclamptic, then an **awake** intubation would be safest. In this case, the risk of severe hypertension and intracranial hemorrhage argue against an **awake** intubation. Perform a rapid sequence induction.

FRC is reduced by both **obesity** and **full-term pregnancy**. Oxygen consumption is up secondary to **full-term pregnancy**. The time to arterial desaturation after preoxygenation (don't forget preoxygenation!) will be very short indeed. The risk of aspiration is **increased** from obesity and pregnancy.

elective C-section The patient is NPO but the stomach is still **full.** Given the **aspiration** risk, administer a nonparticulate antacid. Cimetidine, ranitidine, and metoclopramide have not been reported to cause adverse effects on the fetus; however, long-term effects are **unknown.** I would not give these drugs. [This is a controversial answer.]

hypertension and proteinuria Pre-eclampsia, pre-eclampsia, pre-eclampsia! She needs **coags, a recent platelet count, and fluid** before an epidural is placed. If she has oliguria unresponsive to fluid administration, she needs a **central line.** If there are signs of congestive heart failure or decreased oxygenation (possible pulmonary edema), a **pulmonary artery catheter** should be placed. She may be difficult to intubate due to upper airway and vocal cord **edema.** Renal failure may be associated with this condition. **Intracranial hemorrhage** with severe hypertension can be a fatal complication.

magnesium Can cause a floppy child. The floppiness can be reversed in the newborn with time or with **calcium.**

BP 145/95 Severe pre-eclampsia (minimum BP 160/110) warrants an arterial line. Unless this patient has other signs of severe pre-eclampsia (**CNS disturbances, visual changes, 4+ proteinuria, severe oliguria**), she does not need an arterial line.

CASE 4 *(preop/intraop/postop approach)*

obesity

A 34-year-old, 122 kg male is scheduled for an urgent cholecystectomy. He has diabetes, treated with 40 units of NPH daily. He describes an allergic reaction during a dental extraction. BP 150/90; HR 80; WBC 32,000; T 39.5°C; glucose 350.

PREOP

1. **Labs** Sample blood gases to determine both baseline _____ and to rule out resting _hypercapnia_. The blood gases will also reveal if the patient is acidotic (ketotic) from his diabetes.

Given this degree of obesity, the patient may be chronically _hypoxic_ or even pickwickian. FEV_1 and FVC may also be needed if the patient has a history of dyspnea on exertion. A restrictive pattern (normal FEV_1/FVC, low FEV_1, low FVC) will probably be seen. You can rule out treatable, reversible obstructive disease with an evaluation of the $MMEF_{25-75}$ with and without _broncho dilator_ if there is time.

Compare new and old _EKg's_ to help evaluate the effect of diabetes on the heart. The history may be negative since these patients are particularly prone to silent _ischemia_.

Creatinine and BUN are needed to evaluate the end-organ effect of _DIAbeTes_ on the kidney.

2. **Consults** The only consult should be with the _Dentist_ in an effort to elucidate the allergic reaction. The board examiners will most likely not give you this information. Be prepared for _Anaphylaxis_ later on in the case.

Preparing for the Anesthesia Orals

You should be able to interpret the PFTs and see if the patient will need postop ___ventilator___.

3. Further medical treatment Start treating the hyperglycemia, conceding that diabetes is hard to control during an ___infection___. Aggressively treat if there is ___ketosis___. Give bronchodilators if there is an element of reversible obstructive pulmonary disease. Consider prophylactic ___NTG___ if the ECG demonstrates silent ischemic heart disease. Consider renal-dose dopamine if there is renal compromise.

INTRAOP

1. Special considerations Morbid obesity has several associated difficulties: difficult ___airway___; difficulty placing lines (the patient may have a passive-aggressive personality); chronic hypoxemia with attendant ___Pickwickian___; hypertension and possible associated left heart dysfunction; markedly decreased time to ___Desaturation___ following preoxygenation (decreased FRC, increased oxygen consumption with obesity and temperature); and increased ___aspiration___ risk. There is a risk of injury to OR personnel when moving the patient.

Diabetes mandates monitoring the blood glucose and acid-base status. To prevent ___ketosis___, treat hyperglycemia with insulin, but *frequently follow glucose levels.* _____ under anesthesia is difficult to diagnose by clinical means alone. If ketosis is present, continue giving insulin and glucose until it is controlled. Normoglycemia is not an indication that diabetic ketoacidosis is under control.

Allergic reaction to a local anesthetic: most likely the patient got toxic from an ___ester___ or an _____ injection of local anesthetic. Prudence would dictate avoiding the ester anesthetics (like procaine), which can precipitate a real allergic reaction.

2. Monitors Place an arterial line for frequent blood gas monitoring and blood glucose determinations. A Foley catheter to monitor volume status will be inadequate since there will be an _osmotic_ diuresis with a blood glucose of 350. A CVP line is necessary. If signs of right heart failure are present, a pulmonary artery catheter should be used. In a patient with ongoing osmotic diuresis, an elevated temperature, and an abdominal infection, _dehydration_ should be expected.

3. Induction   Given the patient's size, perform an _awake_ intubation. If you can't see orally with atraumatic laryngoscopy, use fiberoptic nasal intubation as a backup plan. If you attempt a rapid sequence induction and are unable to intubate, the patient will rapidly _desaturate_. The excessive soft tissue may make mask ventilation difficult and you may end up with an airway catastrophe.

4. Maintenance   Enflurane/oxygen. Don't start nitrous oxide until a blood gas proves you can. Minimize narcotics for two reasons:

   1. Narcotics can cause _biliary spasm_ thus making the intraoperative cholangiogram difficult to interpret.

   2. If the patient is pickwickian, the slightest amount of postoperative respiratory depression may result in respiratory arrest.

5. Emergence   Since the patient had a full stomach, he should be fully awake prior to _extubation_. Given the patient's size and the site of the surgery, postoperative respiratory support may be necessary. Availability of an _____ bed is mandatory.

6. Intraop problems

   a. _Hypoxemia._ As in the earlier stem question, the best technique can still have an adverse outcome. The most likely cause is upper abdominal retraction compressing _basilar_ areas of lung and increasing pulmonary shunting. Patients can silently _aspirate_, even during an awake intubation. This aspiration may manifest intraoperatively as a low pO_2. Also high on the differential will be _pneumothorax_. Ventilating morbidly obese patients requires high inspiratory pressures. Always start by ensuring that you are ventilating to the set volumes and giving 100% oxygen. Hand ventilate. The next step is to listen to the lungs for unequal breath sounds (pneumothorax, _Tension ptx , Endobronchial intub_) and wheezing (bronchospasm, atelectasis, endobronchial intubation, _herniated_ endotracheal tube cuff). Follow these steps by passing a suction catheter down the ET tube (mucus plug, endotracheal tube cuff herniation). Next, ask the surgeons to pause and remove their retractors so that you can _ventilate_ the lungs. Only after these steps should you use PEEP to treat suspected aspiration or continued excessive pulmonary shunting.

b. *Anaphylaxis.* The examiners haven't included a history of allergic reaction in the stem question in order to generate interest from the American Society of Allergists. When hypotension, bronchospasm, and flushing occur, you should be ready. Stop the offending drug and give _100 % O2_. _Epinephrine_ is the drug of choice, preferably titrated to effect unless the patient is coding. Diphenhydramine and steroids should be given for 24 hours following the incident and the patient should be observed for that length of time as well.

POSTOP

1. **Pain**   You walk a tightrope here. Given the patient's size, you do not want to depress _respiration_. If the patient is in severe pain and splinting, however, he will develop _Atelectasis_ and oxygenation will worsen. Intrathecal or epidural narcotics are an attractive choice, providing profound, longlasting pain relief. The threat of late respiratory depression from this treatment, in a patient who may be difficult to reintubate, mandates that the patient be followed in an _ICU_.

2. **Weaning from the ventilator**   If the patient requires postoperative ventilation, he will be ready for extubation when:
   - No sepsis is present
   - He can defend his _airway_
   - His nutrition status is optimized

- He displays adequate pulmonary mechanics (negative inspiratory force ___ > 30 ___, FVC >15 cc/kg, respiratory rate < ___ 30 ___).

Again, fight the urge to take the easy route. Don't just look at what we wrote and say, "Yeah, that's what I was thinking." Wrestle with it yourself. Learning is work. Work at it and it will stick; breeze through it and you'll forget.

~~~~~~~~~~~~~~

PREOP

1. **Labs**   Sample blood gases to determine both baseline **oxygenation** and to rule out resting **hypercapnia**. The blood gases will also reveal if the patient is acidotic (ketotic) from his diabetes.

Given this degree of obesity, the patient may be chronically **hypoxemic** or even pickwickian. FEV_1 and FVC may also be needed if the patient has a history of dyspnea on exertion. A restrictive pattern (normal FEV_1/FVC, low FEV_1, low FVC) will probably be seen. You can rule out treatable, reversible obstructive disease with an evaluation of the $MMEF_{25-75}$ with and without **bronchodilators** if there is time.

Compare new and old **ECG** to help evaluate the effect of diabetes on the heart. The history may be negative since these patients are particularly prone to silent **ischemia**.

Creatinine and BUN are needed to evaluate the end-organ effect of **diabetes** on the kidney.

2. **Consults**   The only consult should be with the **dentist** in an effort to elucidate the allergic reaction. The board examiners will most likely not give you this information. Be prepared for **anaphylaxis** later on in the case.

You should be able to interpret the PFTs and see if the patient will need postop **ventilation**.

3. **Further medical treatment**   Start treating the hyperglycemia, conceding that diabetes is hard to control during an **infection**. Aggressively treat if there is **ketosis**. Give bronchodilators if there is an element of reversible obstructive pulmonary disease. Consider prophylactic **nitroglycerin** if the ECG demonstrates silent ischemic heart disease. Consider renal-dose dopamine if there is renal compromise.

PFTS:

RESTRICTIVE Dx
↓ FEV_1
↓ FRC
~ FEV_1/FVC

obstructive Dx
FEV_1 ↓
FRC ↑
FEV_1/FVC ↓

1. Special considerations   Morbid obesity has several associated difficulties: difficult **airway;** difficulty placing lines (the patient may have a passive-aggressive personality); chronic hypoxemia with attendant **cor pulmonale;** hypertension and possible associated left heart dysfunction; markedly decreased time to **desaturation** following preoxygenation (decreased FRC, increased oxygen consumption with obesity and temperature); and increased **aspiration** risk. There is a risk of injury to OR personnel when moving the patient.

Diabetes mandates monitoring the blood glucose and acid-base status. To prevent **ketosis,** treat hyperglycemia with insulin, but *frequently follow glucose levels.* **Hypoglycemia** under anesthesia is difficult to diagnose by clinical means alone. If ketosis is present, continue giving insulin and glucose until it is controlled. Normoglycemia is not an indication that diabetic ketoacidosis is under control.

Allergic reaction to a local anesthetic: most likely the patient got toxic from an **overdose** or an **intravascular** injection of local anesthetic. Prudence would dictate avoiding the ester anesthetics (like procaine), which can precipitate a real allergic reaction.

2. Monitors   Place an arterial line for frequent blood gas monitoring and blood glucose determinations. A Foley catheter to monitor volume status will be inadequate since there will be an **osmotic** diuresis with a blood glucose of 350. A CVP line is necessary. If signs of right heart failure are present, a pulmonary artery catheter should be used. In a patient with ongoing osmotic diuresis, an elevated temperature, and an abdominal infection, **dehydration** should be expected.

3. Induction   Given the patient's size, perform an **awake** intubation. If you can't see orally with atraumatic laryngoscopy, use fiberoptic nasal intubation as a backup plan. If you attempt a rapid sequence induction and are unable to intubate, the patient will rapidly **desaturate.** The excessive soft tissue may make mask ventilation difficult and you may end up with an airway catastrophe.

4. Maintenance   Enflurane/oxygen. Don't start nitrous oxide until a blood gas proves you can. Minimize narcotics for two reasons:

1. Narcotics can cause **biliary spasm,** thus making the intraoperative cholangiogram difficult to interpret.

2. If the patient is pickwickian, the slightest amount of postoperative respiratory depression may result in respiratory arrest.

5. Emergence   Since the patient had a full stomach, he should be fully awake prior to **extubation.** Given the patient's size and the site of the surgery, postoperative respiratory support may be necessary. Availability of an **ICU** bed is mandatory.

6. Intraop problems

a. *Hypoxemia.* As in the earlier stem question, the best technique can still have an adverse outcome. The most likely cause is upper abdominal retraction compressing **basilar** areas of lung and increasing pulmonary shunting. Patients can silently **aspirate,** even during an awake intubation. This aspiration may manifest intraoperatively as a low pO_2. Also high on the differential will be **pneumothorax.** Ventilating morbidly obese patients requires high inspiratory pressures. Always start by ensuring that you are ventilating to the set volumes and giving 100% oxygen. Hand ventilate. The next step is to listen to the lungs for unequal breath sounds (pneumothorax, **endobronchial intubation**) and wheezing (bronchospasm, atelectasis, endobronchial intubation, **herniated** endotracheal tube cuff). Follow these steps by passing a suction catheter down the ET tube (mucus plug, endotracheal tube cuff herniation). Next, ask the surgeons to pause and remove their retractors so that you can **reinflate** the lungs. Only after these steps should you use PEEP to treat suspected aspiration or continued excessive pulmonary shunting.

b. *Anaphylaxis.* The examiners haven't included a history of allergic reaction in the stem question in order to generate interest from the American Society of Allergists. When hypotension, bronchospasm, and flushing occur, you should be ready. Stop the offending drug and give **100% oxygen. Epinephrine** is the drug of choice, preferably titrated to effect unless the patient is coding. Diphenhydramine and steroids should be given for 24 hours following the incident and the patient should be observed for that length of time as well.

~~~~~~~~~~~~~~~~

POSTOP

1. Pain   You walk a tightrope here. Given the patient's size, you do not want to depress **respiration.** If the patient is in severe pain and splinting, however, he will develop **atelectasis** and oxygenation will worsen. Intrathecal or epidural narcotics are an attractive choice, providing profound, longlasting pain relief. The threat of late respiratory depression from this treatment, in a patient who may be difficult to reintubate, mandates that the patient be followed in an **ICU.**

2. Weaning from the ventilator If the patient requires postoperative ventilation, he will be ready for extubation when:

No sepsis is present
He can defend his **airway**
His nutrition status is optimized
He displays adequate pulmonary mechanics (negative inspiratory force >**30 cm H₂O,** FVC >15 cc/kg, respiratory rate <**30/min**).

CASE 5   *(word/phrase approach)*

A 74-year-old, 75 kg male with <u>urinary obstruction</u> due to benign prostatic hypertrophy is scheduled for <u>transurethral resection of the prostate (TURP)</u>. <u>Five months</u> earlier he sustained a <u>myocardial infarction</u> (MI) and now takes digoxin, isosorbide, nitroglycerin (sublingual, PRN) and warfarin. BP 170/100; HR 100; R 20; ECG shows atrial fib.

urinary obstruction Check ___Bun___ and ___Creatinine___ to see if the obstruction has caused actual renal damage. If the kidney is damaged, check for ___Hyperkalemia___. If the obstruction is not too severe, perhaps the patient can wait a month before the operation. You would prefer to wait until ___>6___ months have passed since the MI.

TURP Think of the major intraop problems inherent with a TURP: ___hypoNatremia___, manifested as mental changes, and bladder ___perforation___, manifested as shoulder pain. Hyponatremia *rarely* requires hypertonic saline. Better to treat with _____ and normal saline, and stop the operation/bladder irrigation.

A general or spinal anesthetic is acceptable. The advantage of a spinal is that you can continually assess mental status.

MI 5 months ago   From 0 to 3 months the perioperative rate of
reinfarction is about _____30 %_____, from 3 to 6 months the rate
is 15%, and beyond 6 months it is _____5 %_____. By placing patients in the ICU for 3 days with invasive monitoring, Rao et al.
significantly reduced the number of postoperative infarctions.
In any study, the mortality from a postop MI is a whopping
_____50%_____.

   With an MI so recent and all the potential fluid absorption
from a TURP, a Swan is mandatory to guide fluid management.

digoxin   Give the digoxin, the patient needs it for _____Heart   rate_____
_____control_____. His ventricular response is too high
as is, and he may need a higher dose. Make sure you check the
potassium. Although it may not matter to anesthetic outcome
($K^+ > 3.1$), it is always best to optimize factors that will decrease a drug's toxicity.

warfarin   Stop the warfarin _____3 days_____ before the operation, place the patient on heparin, and stop the heparin
_____4 hrs_____ before the procedure.

nitro sublingual   Give the patient Nitropaste on call and have him
come to the OR with a little bottle of nitro tabs. Have IV nitroglycerin mixed and in the room.

atrial fib   If the ventricular response becomes so fast intraop
that there is hemodynamic compromise, then emergency
_____Cardioversion_____ may be necessary. The defibrillator
should be on _____synchronous_____ when you discharge
the paddles. Cardioverting a person on digoxin always runs
the risk of ventricular fibrillation or _____asystole_____, but if you
need to cardiovert, you need to cardiovert.

BP 170/100   This blood pressure would not normally cause a cancellation (diastolic cutoff, > _110_ mm Hg). However, the lability associated with inadequately treated hypertension would
make us want to delay this case until the blood pressure could
be brought well under control, in light of the recent _MI_.
There is an increased incidence of ischemia associated with the

expected blood pressure lability. A cardiology consult should be obtained to optimize blood pressure and heart rate control.

HR 100 Check the chart for other heart rates. If there are any above 100, then the heart rate is not adequately controlled. Tachycardia is detrimental to myocardial oxygen supply/demand. Make sure the heart rate does not exceed 100 beats per minute on a monitor. The recorded pulse rate may be much _____slower_____ than the actual rate since not all electrically conducted beats will be felt as a radial pulsation. It may be necessary to _____increase_____ the digoxin dose. A digoxin level is not necessary. The end point of digoxin therapy in atrial fibrillation is _____HR Control_____ or toxicity, not blood levels.

Vital signs are _____VITAL_____!

spinal — level should be TO T6

~~~~~~~~~~~~~~~~~~~~~~

urinary obstruction Check **BUN** and **creatinine** to see if the obstruction has caused actual renal damage. If the kidney is damaged, check for **hyperkalemia.** If the obstruction is not too severe, perhaps the patient can wait a month before the operation. You would prefer to wait until **6** months have passed since the MI.

TURP Think of the major intraop problems inherent with a TURP: **hyponatremia,** manifested as mental changes, and bladder **rupture,** manifested as shoulder pain. Hyponatremia *rarely* requires hypertonic saline. Better to treat with **furosemide** and normal saline, and stop the operation/bladder irrigation.

A general or spinal anesthetic is acceptable. The advantage of a spinal is that you can continually assess mental status.

MI 5 months ago From 0 to 3 months the perioperative rate of reinfarction is about **30%,** from 3 to 6 months the rate is **15%,** and beyond 6 months it is **5%.** By placing patients in the ICU for 3 days with invasive monitoring, Rao et al. significantly reduced the number of postoperative infarctions. In any study, the mortality from a postop MI is a whopping **50%.**

With an MI so recent and all the potential fluid absorption from a TURP, a Swan is mandatory to guide fluid management.

digoxin Give the digoxin, the patient needs it for **heart rate control.** His ventricular response is too high as is, and he may need a higher dose. Make sure you check the potassium. Although it may not matter to anesthetic outcome (K^+ >3.1), it is always best to optimize factors that will decrease a drug's toxicity.

warfarin Stop the warfarin **3 days before** the operation, place the patient on heparin, and stop the heparin **4 hours** before the procedure.

nitro sublingual Give the patient Nitropaste on call and have him come to the OR with a little bottle of nitro tabs. Have IV nitroglycerin mixed and in the room.

atrial fib If the ventricular response becomes so fast intraop that there is hemodynamic compromise, then emergency **cardioversion** may be necessary. The defibrillator should be on **synchronous** when you discharge the paddles. Cardioverting a person on digoxin always runs the risk of ventricular fibrillation or **asystole,** but if you need to cardiovert, you need to cardiovert.

BP 170/100 This blood pressure would not normally cause a cancellation (diastolic cutoff, >**110** mm Hg). However, the lability associated with inadequately treated hypertension would make us want to delay this case until the blood pressure could be brought well under control, in light of the recent **MI.** There is an increased incidence of ischemia associated with the expected blood pressure lability. A cardiology consult should be obtained to optimize blood pressure and heart rate control.

HR 100 Check the chart for other heart rates. If there are any above 100, then the heart rate is not adequately controlled. Tachycardia is detrimental to myocardial oxygen supply/demand. Make sure the heart rate does not exceed 100 beats per minute on a monitor. The recorded pulse rate may be much **slower** than the actual rate since not all electrically conducted beats will be felt as a radial pulsation. It may be necessary to **increase** the digoxin dose. A digoxin level is not necessary. The end point of digoxin therapy in atrial fibrillation is **heart rate control** or toxicity, not blood levels.

Vital signs are **vital!**

CASE 6 (*preop/intraop/postop approach*)

A 44-year-old, 70 kg male is admitted for thoracotomy for carcinoma of the right lung. He has a long history of smoking. He sustained a myocardial infarction (MI) 5 months ago and now takes propranolol, 80 mg/day. You detect a left-sided carotid bruit. BP 140/80; P 55; R 18; T 37°C.

PREOP

(handwritten margin note:)
Predicting Tolerance For Pneum:

$FEV_1 > 2L$

$MVV > 50\% \text{ pred.}$

$RV/TLC < 50\%$

IF Any oF these Are Abn
↓
Split Function Studies

1. **Labs**   Order __PFT's__ (the examiners are sure to ask which ones—see Chapter 9 if you don't remember) to ensure that the patient can remain ventilator independent after a pneumonectomy. Even if a ___Lobectomy___ is planned, a ___pneumonectomy___ may be performed due to extension of the tumor or intraoperative ___bleeding___. Also rule out reversible obstruction from reactive airways disease. Check ___Blood gas___ on room air. The presence of resting ___hypercapnia___ also determines if the patient can tolerate a pneumonectomy.

Compare old and new ECGs. Why is the patient bradycardic? Are there any new signs of myocardial damage since the MI 5 months ago? Don't ask the examiners the questions. Say, "I would check that the patient is in sinus bradycardia attributable to good beta-blockade and that the ECG shows no new changes."

Obtain a chest x-ray to rule out ___pneumonia___/ that can be associated with lung cancer.

2. **Consults**   A neurology consult is unnecessary if the carotid bruit is ___assymptomatic___. If the carotid bruit is symptomatic (TIA, stroke), then neurology should be asked the *specific* question, "Patient has a symptomatic carotid bruit. What is the best method of evaluating this bruit?" If the workup reveals an operative lesion, a carotid endarterectomy should be planned prior to resecting the lung lesion.

(handwritten note bottom right:)
Bronchogenic Ca — metabolic manifestations:
1) myasthenia gravis   6) peripheral Neuritis
2) Cushing's Synd
3) Carcinoid Synd
4) ↑ Cal
5) Hyponatremia - 2° IADH

Get a pulmonary consult if there are abnormal PFTs that might be amenable to therapy. Then ask the *specific* questions: "___is this pt. optimized for surgery___? Is the bronchospasm under ideal control? Does the patient have a concurrent infection amenable to antibiotics?"

Get a cardiology consult and ask the *specific* questions: "Is the patient's ___cardiac___ therapy optimized? What is the patient's ___ventricular___ function? Does the patient require further workup of his angina? Specifically, does this patient need ___card. cath___?"

A note on all these consults: On the actual exam, the examiners will tell you, "Cardiology saw the man and said 'Cleared for spinal'"—that is to say, the consults will not help you. You yourself should be able to answer the questions posed to the consultants. Or be prepared to make an assumption that will help you: "Assuming that further workup revealed no left ventricular dysfunction, then I would. . . ." You can help yourself.

3. Further medical therapy If reversible airway obstruction from reactive airways disease is present, you must weigh the benefits of treatment against the effects of such treatment on the heart. A therapeutic ___theophylline___ level and round-the-clock ___beta___ inhalation treatment may cause unwanted tachycardia.

Given the recent myocardial infarction, optimize antianginal therapy.

INTRAOP

1. Special considerations A double-lumen tube is nice but not _____. Double-lumen tubes are absolutely indicated when you want to isolate one lung from the other, such as:

- ___Abscess / Alveolar Proteinosis___, where you lavage one lung;
- ___Hemorrhage___, where you bleed into one lung;
- ___Purulent infect.___, where you gross out one lung;

- _____*Broncho Pleural Fistula*_____, where you blow off one lung

2. **Monitors**   A-line for _____*Blood gas Analysis*_____.
A pulmonary artery catheter is indicated since there has been a _____*cardiac insult*_____. An early indication of ischemia will be a rise in _____*wedge*_____ pressure with no change or a fall in cardiac output. Placement can be a little problematic if a right _____ is performed. You will have to pull the _____*cath*_____ back when the right pulmonary artery is clamped. Even with a clamped pulmonary artery, the cardiac outputs will probably be accurate.

A real brainbuster of a question for thoracotomy stem questions is, "What happens to _____*CVP*_____ and _____*wedge Press*_____ when the chest is open?" Give up? They ought to stay the same as long as you take your readings at end-expiration. How about, "What happens to the PA readings when the lung is down and you are looking at a pulmonary artery with lots of

_____?"

The pressure readings from the PA catheter may not change if an _____ fluid column remains open between the left atrium and the balloon, which is wedged in a small pulmonary artery. (_____
may interfere with this assumption.)

_____ would be useful, especially for detecting a _____. Disconnects can occur easily with a double-lumen tube.

Place a _____ line to help assess volume status.
3. **Induction**   Because of the patient's cardiac disease, avoid _____*Tachycardia*_____ and avoid extremes in _____*BP*_____.
A slow induction combining IV (narcotics and lidocaine) and _____*induction*_____ agents (tailored to pre-existing myocardial dysfunction, if present) to _____*blunt response to*_____ _____*intubation*_____ would be best. Ensure complete _____*muscular Relaxation*_____ before in-

79   *Sample Questions*

strumenting the airway. Otherwise, the double-lumen tube is a bit tough to place at times.

4. Maintenance Enflurane/oxygen supplemented with _____NARCOTICS_____. Halothane and isoflurane are also acceptable. If you believe in _____corn. steal_____ (we don't), then you may want to avoid isoflurane.

5. Emergence Some practitioners extubate right from the double-lumen tube, others _____switch to single lumen Tube_____ then extubate from there. In either case, extubate the patient as soon as possible to avoid exposing the _____ to _____.

Tachycardia and hypertension are likely to accompany _____Extubation_____. Treat with hydralazine, metoprolol, esmolol, or labetolol (_____Verapamil_____ if bronchospasm is a concern) to minimize these adverse hemodynamic effects.

6. Intraop problems

a. _____Hypoxemia_____ is possible when you deflate one lung. Listen to the chest to make sure you have not extubated the patient (unlikely with the long double-lumen tube), turn on _____100 % O₂_____ (of course), _____hand vent._____ (of course), _____Pull The Tube back_____ (you may have occluded the upper lobe by advancing the tube too far), suction, try _____CPAP_____ on the lung you are not ventilating and then _____peep_____ on the lung you are ventilating. Finally, don't _____Kill The PT_____ to prove a point. If at any time the patient's saturation drops to below _90_ %, _____ventilate/Reinflate_____ both lungs and tell the surgeons to cool their jets while you and a colleague figure out what to do. A fiberoptic bronchoscope to visualize the position of the double-lumen tube is an excellent diagnostic device.

b. *The lung won't deflate.* Check your _____Tube_____, you may have dropped the _____. _____ the tube (remember to deflate the cuffs before you slide the tube around). You may have slipped all the way up the trachea and popped the endotracheal tube down the wrong pipe. In this

case, _____
_____, then they can direct the endotracheal tube down the correct passage. _____ to confirm the correct position may also help. If all else fails, the surgeons can do the operation with _____. The surgeons will have to place special _____ in the field.

   c. *CPR.* Don't forget that the _____ and that _____ is an immediate recourse. Expect these thoracotomy patients to code sometime during your exam.

POSTOP

1. **Pain** __*Intrathecal*__ and __*Epidural*__ narcotics would provide good pain relief for this exquisitely painful procedure. Infusion of a local anesthetic through an __*Epidural*__ catheter would also be acceptable. (As mentioned earlier, don't bring up unfamiliar topics. If you don't know about intrapleural catheters, don't mention them.) PCA is also a fine choice. IM and IV narcotics, although antiquated (you can tell we live in an ivory tower), are still effective if you don't know anything else.

2. **ICU** __*All pts s/p Thoracotomy need to be*__ __*in ICU*__.

3. **Catastrophic hypotension** A suture on the __*Pulm*__ __*Artery*__ could have come off. After a pneumonectomy, the heart can __*herniate*__ through a defect in the pericardium and cause immediate _____ of the great vessels. A chest tube may malfunction and cause a

_____.

   Therapy in all cases consists of fluids, _____
_____
_____
_____
_____
_____.

Less info given here—you should be working a little harder.

Sample Questions

PREOP

1. Labs Order **PFTs** (the examiners are sure to ask which ones—see Chapter 9 if you don't remember) to ensure that the patient can remain ventilator independent after a pneumonectomy. Even if a **lobectomy** is planned, a **pneumonectomy** may be performed due to extension of the tumor or intraoperative **bleeding.** Also rule out reversible obstruction from reactive airways disease. Check an **arterial blood gas** on room air. The presence of resting **hypercapnia** also determines if the patient can tolerate a pneumonectomy.

Compare old and new ECGs. Why is the patient bradycardic? Are there any new signs of myocardial damage since the MI 5 months ago? Don't ask the examiners the questions. Say, "I would check that the patient is in sinus bradycardia attributable to good beta-blockage and that the ECG shows no new changes."

Obtain a chest x-ray to rule out **pneumonia** that can be associated with lung cancer.

2. Consults A neurology consult is unnecessary if the carotid bruit is **asymptomatic.** If the carotid bruit is symptomatic (TIA, stroke), then neurology should be asked the *specific* question, "Patient has a symptomatic carotid bruit. What is the best method of evaluating this bruit?" If the workup reveals an operative lesion, a carotid endarterectomy should be planned prior to resecting the lung lesion.

Get a pulmonary consult if there are abnormal PFTs that might be amenable to therapy. Then ask the *specific* questions: "**Is this patient in optimal condition for surgery?** Is the bronchospasm under ideal control? Does the patient have a concurrent infection amenable to antibiotics?"

Get a cardiology consult and ask the *specific* questions: "Is the patient's **antianginal** therapy optimized? What is the patient's **ventricular** function? Does the patient require further workup of his angina? Specifically, does this patient need **catheterization?**"

A note on all these consults: On the actual exam, the examiners will tell you, "Cardiology saw the man and said 'Cleared for spinal' "—that is to say, the consults will not help you. You yourself should be able to answer the questions posed to the consultants. Or be prepared to make an assumption that will help you: "Assuming that further workup revealed no left ventricular dysfunction, then I would. . . ." You can help yourself.

3. Further medical therapy If reversible airway obstruction from reactive airways disease is present, you must weigh the benefits of treatment against the effects of such treatment on the heart. A therapeutic **theophylline** level and round-the-clock **beta** inhalation treatment may cause unwanted tachycardia.

Given the recent myocardial infarction, optimize antianginal therapy.

INTRAOP

1. Special considerations A double-lumen tube is nice but not **absolutely indicated.** Double-lumen tubes are absolutely indicated when you want to isolate one lung from the other, such as:

Alveolar proteinosis, where you lavage one lung;
Hemorrhage, where you bleed into one lung;
Purulence, where you gross out one lung;
Bronchopleural fistula, where you blow off one lung.

2. Monitors A-line for **frequent blood gases.**

A pulmonary artery catheter is indicated since there has been a **recent MI.** An early indication of ischemia will be a rise in **wedge** pressure with no change or a fall in cardiac output. Placement can be a little problematic if a right **pneumonectomy** is performed. You will have to pull the **PA catheter** back when the right pulmonary artery is clamped. Even with a clamped pulmonary artery, the cardiac outputs will probably be accurate.

A real brainbuster of a question for thoracotomy stem questions is, "What happens to **CVP** and **Swan numbers** when the chest is open?" Give up? They ought to stay the same as long as you take your readings at end-expiration. How about, "What happens to the PA readings when the lung is down and you are looking at a pulmonary artery with lots of **hypoxic pulmonary vasoconstriction?**" The pressure readings from the PA catheter may not change if an **uninterrupted** fluid column remains open between the left atrium and the balloon, which is wedged in a small pulmonary artery. (**Hypoxic pulmonary vasoconstriction** may interfere with this assumption.)

End-tidal CO_2 would be useful, especially for detecting a **disconnect.** Disconnects can occur easily with a double-lumen tube.

Place a **Foley** line to help assess volume status.

3. Induction Because of the patient's cardiac disease, avoid **tachycardia** and avoid extremes in **blood pressure.** A slow induction combining IV (narcotics and lidocaine) and **inhalation** agents (tailored to pre-existing myocardial dysfunction, if present) to **blunt sympathetic response to intubation** would be best. Ensure complete **neuromuscular relaxation** before instrumenting the airway. Otherwise, the double-lumen tube is a bit tough to place at times.

4. Maintenance   Enflurane/oxygen supplemented with **narcotics.** Halothane and isoflurane are also acceptable. If you believe in **coronary steal** (we don't), then you may want to avoid isoflurane.

5. Emergence   Some practitioners extubate right from the double-lumen tube, others **always change to a single-lumen tube** then extubate from there. In either case, extubate the patient as soon as possible to avoid exposing the **fresh stump** to **positive airways pressure.**

Tachycardia and hypertension are likely to accompany **emergence.** Treat with hydralazine, metoprolol, esmolol, or labetolol (**verapamil** if bronchospasm is a concern) to minimize these adverse hemodynamic effects.

6. Intraop problems

a. **Hypoxemia** is possible when you deflate one lung. Listen to the chest to make sure you have not extubated the patient (unlikely with the long double-lumen tube), turn on **100% O$_2$** (of course), **hand ventilate** (of course), **pull the tube back** (you may have occluded the upper lobe by advancing the tube too far), suction, try **CPAP** on the lung you are not ventilating and then **PEEP** on the lung you are ventilating. Finally, don't **kill the patient** to prove a point. If at any time the patient's saturation drops to below **90%, reinflate** both lungs and tell the surgeons to cool their jets while you and a colleague figure out what to do. A fiberoptic bronchoscope to visualize the position of the double-lumen tube is an excellent diagnostic device.

b. *The lung won't deflate.* Check your **cuffs,** you may have dropped the **wrong lung. Advance** the tube (remember to deflate the cuffs before you slide the tube around). You may have slipped all the way up the trachea and popped the endotracheal tube down the wrong pipe. In this case, **enlist the surgeons' help and have them feel the bronchus for a balloon,** then they can direct the endotracheal tube down the correct passage. **Fiberoptic scoping** to confirm the correct position may also help. If all else fails, the surgeons can do the operation with **both lungs inflated.** The surgeons will have to place special **retractors** in the field.

c. *CPR.* Don't forget that the **chest is open** and that **open heart**

massage is an immediate recourse. Expect these thoracotomy patients to code sometime during your exam.

POSTOP

1. Pain **Intrathecal** and **epidural** narcotics would provide good pain relief for this exquisitely painful procedure. Infusion of a local anesthetic through an **intrapleural** catheter would also be acceptable. (As mentioned earlier, don't bring up unfamiliar topics. If you don't know about intrapleural catheters, don't mention them.) PCA is also a fine choice. IM and IV narcotics, although antiquated (you can tell we live in an ivory tower), are still effective if you don't know anything else.

2. ICU **Any patient post-thoracotomy needs ICU care.**

3. Catastrophic hypotension A suture on the **pulmonary artery** could have come off. After a pneumonectomy, the heart can **herniate** through a defect in the pericardium and cause immediate **torsion** of the great vessels. A chest tube may malfunction and cause a **tension pneumothorax.**

Therapy in all cases consists of fluids, **hand ventilation, intubation if necessary, calls for help, a quick listen to the chest to check for pneumothorax, and a return trip to the operating room as quickly as possible. If the heart has herniated, (rare) a change in position might help.**

CASE 7 *(word/phrase approach)*

A 67-year-old, 65 kg female is admitted for resection of a cecal carcinoma. She has a long history of alcoholism and appears inebriated on admission. She has a bottle of Mad Dog 20/20 on her bedside table and offers you a swig. Her liver is enlarged and she has ascites. BP 130/90; P 78; R 18; Hgb 11.2; serum protein 5.4; albumin 2.1; Na+ 132; SGOT 400; T 37.5°C.

alcoholism with all the trimmings Proceeding on an elective case with an SGOT out the roof is folly. _Repeat SGOT if ↑ — get GI consult. Document it._ If the SGOT stays high or goes higher, you need a ___GI consult___ to ask the *specific* questions, "Is the elevated SGOT due to a chronic

or an acute problem? Will the hepatic dysfunction resolve? If
not, _____
_____
_____?"

The decreased *protein, albumin, and sodium* all tell you
that the patient has an _____.
The response to _____ will be
increased.

Neuromuscular blockers need to be given in ↑ Doses_____
initially to overcome the increased _vol. of Dist._____
associated with an _____. These
patients then need lower subsequent doses due to _____
_____. _Sux_____

action will be slightly prolonged due to the decreased pseudocholinesterase. _Atracurium_____ is the only drug whose
subsequent doses will not need to be decreased since _____
_it is degraded by Hoffman Degradation_____
_____
_____.

Check coagulation parameters. Patients with liver disease
_ha_____.
Check _____ since the typical cirrhotic has
an enlarged __Spleen_____ and sequesters _platelets_____.

Check the glucose. ___glycogen_____ stores are depleted and hypoglycemia is a concern.

Check the baseline blood gases and the chest x-ray. The
pulmonary function of an alcoholic is affected by _Enlarging___
_Abdomen 2° to Ascites_____
_____
_____.

Which anesthetic is best for the patient with liver disease?
Liver blood flow decreases to the same extent with _____,
_____, and _____ anesthesia. Halothane is
_____, even in patients with cirrhosis,
but most practitioners would not use halothane. Any postopera-

tive deterioration in liver function _____
_____. Essentially, titration of any anesthetic is
acceptable for these patients as long as ___↓ Blood Flow to___
___Liver___ is anticipated.

ascites Ascites may exert so much pressure on the abdomen that
___IT compromises Pulm. Function___.
The functional residual capacity (FRC) then ___↓___
and hypoxemia results, especially in the ___supine___ position. ___Drain Ascites___ in such a case. Do not drain the
ascites if ventilation is unimpaired. (This is a favorite question
of the examiners.)

The presence of ascites makes this patient a ___Full___
___stomach___ case. The possibility of rapid desaturation
(decreased FRC) even with preoxygenation makes a ___RAPID___
___sequence___ induction a little risky. Don't take chances
on the boards. Optimize the patient's ___coagulation___
status, give a topical, and proceed with an awake intubation. A
rapid sequence can then be your backup plan. If the examiners
can complicate your initial plan, they will do so. Failing with an
awake intubation and adapting with a rapid sequence will probably satisfy your examiners and leave you at ease. Failing with a
rapid sequence induction and dealing with ___hypoxemia___,
___Aspiration___, and ___coding PT___ in
the first few minutes of your exam is not a great confidence
builder. People with conservative, safe approaches pass the
exam.

Mad Dog 20/20 ___Alcohol Ingestion___ reduces
the anesthetic requirements. If the patient is not acutely intoxicated, the ___history___ of alcohol with other seda-
tive/hypnotics will increase drug requirements.

DTs If full-blown DTs develop, the patient has about a ___15 %___
chance of dying. That is about the same odds as Russian
roulette with a six-chamber pistol. Start treatment with
___benzo's___ to prevent development of DTs. Anes-

87

thetic drugs will usually prevent the occurrence of DTs in the OR, but postoperatively ___*sympathetic discharge*___ and ___*Emergence Delerium*___ should set off a flashing red light to consider DTs. Prevention is better than treatment. ___*Thiamine*___ and ___*VIT K*___ should have been given IM upon admission to the hospital. On the boards, take nothing for granted.

Know how to evaluate postoperative delayed awakening and postoperative delirium. Approach this problem just as you would any other problem in anesthesia. First, _____ _____. Check ABC (airway, breathing, circulation). Administer ___*O₂*___, check blood gases and pulse oximetry readings (if available) in the recovery room. Look at the vital signs and make sure the patient is _____. Do a finger stick for _____. Then start down the differential in an organized fashion: *drugs; metabolic; neurologic.*

Drugs: For this patient, list the most likely causes in each category first. All preop, intraop, and postop drugs can be responsible, especially given the expectation of _____ _____. _____. Consider if the patient has been treated for DTs (_____) or hasn't (_____). Was _____ given before dextrose was administered to this glycogen-depleted alcoholic?

Metabolic: _____ _____ _____ must be ruled out by checking ABC. _____, _____, and _____ (starting with a hemoglobin of only 11) are secondary possibilities. _____ _____ _____ can be considered way down the list.

Preparing for the Anesthesia Orals

Neurologic: Has the patient seized and is she now _____ _____? You could consider _____ and _____ _____ here. Was there an ischemic insult to the brain intraoperatively with _____, _____, or _____? In a recently admitted alcoholic, consider _____.

Hgb 11.2 The liver is already damaged. Set a transfusion limit for this patient at a hematocrit of _____. You must try to _____ (the examiners like to hear that phrase) to the liver. An A-line is a reasonable, defensible monitoring option. You will need to check the _____ frequently, and an A-line would serve to monitor perfusion pressure to the liver.

Do you need a CVP line, too? Have a low threshold for placing one if the urine output decreases below _____. Perioperative renal failure is terrible anytime. Essentially, _____ syndrome equals death. Maintaining adequate _____ is the least you can do. By now, you should know that if the examiners ask you about a pulmonary artery catheter, you should answer, "_____ _____ _____ _____ _____."

Getting a little harder to read our minds?

~~~~~~~~~~~~~~~~

alcoholism with all the trimmings Proceeding on an elective case with an SGOT out the roof is folly. **Document a falling SGOT before proceeding.** If the SGOT stays high or goes higher, you need a **GI evaluation** to ask the *specific* questions, "Is the elevated SGOT due to a chronic or an acute problem? Will the hepatic dysfunction resolve? If not, **are there any interventions that will optimize the patient's liver function prior to surgery?**"

The decreased *protein, albumin, and sodium* all tell you that the patient has an **excess of total body water.** The response to **protein-bound drugs** will be increased.

Neuromuscular blockers need to be given in **larger doses** initially to overcome the increased **volume of distribution** associated with an **excess of total body water.** These patients then need lower subsequent doses due to **decreased hepatic clearance. Succinylcholine** action will be slightly prolonged due to the decreased pseudocholinesterase. **Atracurium** is the only drug whose subsequent doses will not need to be decreased since it **utilizes two nonhepatic elimination pathways: pH-mediated Hoffman degradation, and enzymatic destruction by plasma nonspecific esterases.**

Check coagulation parameters. Patients with liver disease **may not produce adequate coagulation factors.**

Check **platelets** since the typical cirrhotic has an enlarged **spleen** and sequesters **platelets.**

Check the glucose. **Glycogen** stores are depleted and hypoglycemia is a concern.

Check the baseline blood gases and the chest x-ray. The pulmonary function of an alcoholic is affected by **the presence of right-to-left shunts, ascitic compression of basilar lung regions, and acute or chronic pulmonary aspiration.**

Which anesthetic is best for the patient with liver disease? Liver blood flow decreases to the same extent with **general, spinal,** and **epidural** anesthesia. Halothane is **not contraindicated,** even in patients with cirrhosis, but most practitioners would not use halothane. Any postoperative deterioration in liver function **might be attributed to the halothane.** Essentially, titration of any anesthetic is acceptable for these patients as long as **the prolonged action of drugs** is anticipated.

ascites   Ascites may exert so much pressure on the abdomen that **excursion of the diaphragm is impaired.** The functional residual capacity (FRC) then **decreases** and hypoxemia results, especially in the **supine** position. **Drain the ascites** in such a case. Do not drain the ascites if ventilation is unimpaired. (This is a favorite question of the examiners.)

The presence of ascites makes this patient a **full stomach case.** The possibility of rapid desaturation (decreased FRC) even with preoxygenation makes a **rapid sequence** induction a little risky. Don't take chances on the boards. Optimize the patient's **coagulation** status, give a topical, and proceed with an awake intubation. A rapid sequence can then be your backup plan. If the examiners can complicate your initial plan, they will do so. Failing with an awake intubation and adapting with a rapid sequence will probably satisfy your examiners and leave you at ease. Failing with a rapid sequence induction and dealing with **hypoxemia, aspiration,** and **a coding patient** in the first few minutes of your exam is not a great confidence builder. People with conservative, safe approaches pass the exam.

Mad Dog 20/20   **Acute alcoholic intoxication** reduces the anesthetic requirements. If the patient is not acutely intoxicated, the **cross-tolerance** of alcohol with other sedative/hypnotics will increase drug requirements.

DTs   If full-blown DTs develop, the patient has about a **15%** chance of dying. That is about the same odds as Russian roulette with a 6-chamber pistol. Start treatment with **benzodiazepines** to prevent development of DTs. Anesthetic drugs will usually prevent the occurrence of DTs in the OR, but postoperatively **high sympathetic tone** and "**emergence delirium**" should set off a flashing red light to consider DTs. Prevention is better than treatment. **Thiamine** and **vitamin K** should have been given IM upon admission to the hospital. On the boards, take nothing for granted.

Know how to evaluate postoperative delayed awakening and postoperative delirium. Approach this problem just as you would any other problem in anesthesia. First, **rule out life-threatening causes.** Check ABC (airway, breathing, circulation). Administer **supplemental oxygen,** check blood gases and pulse oximetry readings (if available) in the recovery room. Look at the vital signs and make sure the patient is **perfusing her noggin.** Do a finger stick for **glucose.** Then start down the differential in an organized fashion: *drugs; metabolic; neurologic.*

Drugs: For this patient, list the most likely causes in each category first. All preop, intraop, and postop drugs can be responsible, especially given the expectation of **reduced metabolism of anesthetics and neuromuscular blockers.** Consider if the patient has been treated for DTs (**too much Librium**) or hasn't (**hallucinations**). Was **thiamine** given before dextrose was administered to this glycogen-depleted alcoholic?

Metabolic: **Hypoxia, hypercapnia, low blood pressure,** and **hypoglycemia** must be ruled out by checking ABC. **Hyponatremia, ammonia with hepatic encephalopathy,** and **severe anemia** (starting with a hemoglobin of only 11) are secondary possibilities. **Adrenal and thy-**

roid problems, **malignant hyperthermia, hypocalcemia,** and **hypermagnesemia** can be considered way down the list.

Neurologic: Has the patient seized and is she now **postictal**? You could consider **DTs** and **Korsakoff's psychosis** here. Was there an ischemic insult to the brain intraoperatively with **hypotension, hemorrhage,** or **hypoxia**? In a recently admitted alcoholic, consider **subdural hematoma.**

Hgb 11.2 The liver is already damaged. Set a transfusion limit for this patient at a hematocrit of **30.** You must try to **optimize oxygen delivery** (the examiners like to hear that phrase) to the liver. An A-line is a reasonable, defensible monitoring option. You will need to check the **hematocrit** frequently, and an A-line would serve to monitor perfusion pressure to the liver.

Do you need a CVP line, too? Have a low threshold for placing one if the urine output decreases below **0.5 ml/kg/hr.** Perioperative renal failure is terrible anytime. Essentially, **hepatorenal** syndrome equals death. Maintaining adequate **preload** is the least you can do. By now, you should know that if the examiners ask you about a pulmonary artery catheter, you should answer, **"If the urine output doesn't respond to an adequate CVP, then a PA catheter would be warranted in order to document adequate left-sided filling pressures and to guide ionotropic support if the cardiac output is inadequate."**

Disagree with something? Find a better answer in your textbook? Good.

CASE 8 *(preop/intraop/postop approach)*

A 7-week-old, 5 kg boy with communicating hydrocephalus is admitted for placement of a ventriculoperitoneal (VP) shunt. He has been fed IV for 3 days. A 21-gauge "butterfly" is in place on the hand and it appears infiltrated. P 110; T 37.6°C; R 30; Hgb 9.

Screw on your thinking cap. The clues thin out (as does the need for boldface type in our answers).

PREOP

1. Labs

Hematocrit: ↓ Hgb

Glucose: No glucose containing solutions ? ↑ Icp

Gestational age: premature infant ↑ incidence

Sequential weights, urine output, and *physical exam:*

2. Consults A chat with the pediatrician and

3. Further therapy None needed unless

INTRAOP
1. Special considerations
Dehydration:

Heat:

Airway:

Increased intracranial pressure:

Preparing for the Anesthesia Orals

Retrolental fibroplasia:

2. Monitors

3. Induction   Pentothal IV induction with vecuronium and immediate hyperventilation is best if the patient has a _____. Gentle (fat chance) awake laryngoscopy may be indicated if _____ _____. Remember that _____ don't work too well in kids this age. ___KeTAmine___ should be avoided since ICP rises with this agent.

4. Maintenance   Inhaled agents ___↑ Icp-___ _____. Thus, maintenance would be with ___Iso___/air/oxygen. Hyperventilation monitored by end-tidal CO_2 _____ _____.

Heavy-duty narcotics in this age group ___mAy induce___ ___severe Resp Depression___ _____.

Nitrous oxide is also an acceptable adjunct in this case. The effect of nitrous oxide on ICP is ___slight___.

Which circuit will you use?_____

_____

_____

_____.

5. **Emergence** _____.

6. **Intraop problems**

    a. *Dropping oxygen saturation:*

    b. *Bucking on the tube* in spite of neuromuscular relaxation:

POSTOP

    1. Apnea

2. Stridor Small children have small, easily obstructed airways.

The envelope, please.

~~~~~~~~~~~~~~~~~~~

PREOP

   1. Labs

Hematocrit: Although big-time blood loss is not anticipated, this patient may be chronically ill (as chronic as you can get in 7 weeks) and malnourished. Both these factors may account for the anemia. The hemoglobin should not be this low until 3 to 6 months of age. Transfusion is a toss-up. Some areas of the brain may have decreased oxygen delivery due to an increased ICP, and maintaining a hemoglobin of 10 in the perioperative period could be defended. It would be equally OK to defend holding off transfusion because of the risk of hepatitis.

Glucose: A normal 7-week-old infant is unlikely to develop hypoglycemia in the perioperative period, but this child may have low glycogen and body fat stores. Hypoglycemia is a threat to this child.

Gestational age: Not technically lab data. It is important for determining the child's risk for retrolental fibroplasia. A child with developmental abnormalities may be premature or have other associated abnormalities.

Sequential weights, urine output, and *physical exam:* These combined data will clue you in to the patient's fluid status. On the physical exam the skin color, mucous membranes, and heart rate need to be assessed. Sunken fontanelles will not be present with hydrocephalus. The examiners are *sure* to ask how you would evaluate the fluid status prior to coming to the OR (Review Chapter 15, Table 4).

2. Consults   A chat with the pediatrician and parents will land a lot of valuable information. Pediatricians are always so nice, it's a pleasure to talk over the case with them. Changes in behavior, lethargy, or other signs of increased intracranial pressure will be important to elicit.

3. Further therapy   None needed unless the patient has signs of dehydration.

INTRAOP

1. Special considerations

Dehydration: Again, look for clinical signs of dehydration. If the child's IV line has been infiltrated, he may have been NPO for a long time and so may be dehydrated.

Heat: Small children have large surface-to-volume ratios. Therefore heat the room, warm fluids, use radiant warmers, and keep the child well wrapped.

Airway: Hydrocephalic children can have huge heads, making intubation difficult.

Increased intracranial pressure: The procedure itself indicates that increased ICP is a concern. Awake intubation is contraindicated with increased ICP. But so is losing the airway. Hypoxia and hypercapnia don't exactly decrease the ICP. An inhalation induction with its concomitant hypercapnia and cerebral vascular dilation is contraindicated if there are signs of increased ICP. If the airway is normal, an IV induction is the best choice with increased ICP. Placing an IV line may cause crying and increase the ICP, but if the child is awake enough to cry for an IV insertion he probably doesn't have a high enough ICP to suffer a brainstem herniation anyway.

Retrolental fibroplasia: Up to the gestational age of 44 weeks, infants are susceptible to retrolental fibroplasia if exposed to increased FIO_2. If this infant is less than 44 weeks' gestational age, then keep the oxygen *saturation* in the 90% to 95% range to avoid oxygen toxicity. The whole retrolental fibroplasia picture is much more complex than this simple description. Other factors such as overall health, positive-pressure ventilation, hypotension, and degree of immaturity all come into play.

Preparing for the Anesthesia Orals

2. Monitors   Pulse oximeter, BP cuff, ECG, end-tidal CO_2, breath sounds, FIO_2, temperature. In other words, round up the usual suspects.

3. Induction   Pentothal IV induction with vecuronium and immediate hyperventilation is best if the patient has a **normal airway.** Gentle (fat chance) awake laryngoscopy may be indicated if **the large head makes you think that you will have a difficult airway.** Remember that **cricothyrotomies** don't work too well in kids this age. **Ketamine** should be avoided since ICP rises with this agent.

4. Maintenance   Inhaled agents **increase ICP—halothane the most, isoflurane the least.** Thus, maintenance would be with **isoflurane**/air/ oxygen. Hyperventilation monitored by end-tidal CO_2 **would be appropriate to help decrease ICP.** Heavy-duty narcotics in this age group **may result in unpredictable respiratory depression, so minimize the use of these IV agents.**

Nitrous oxide is also an acceptable adjunct in this case. The effect of nitrous oxide on ICP is **slight.**

Which circuit will you use? **A Jackson-Reese or Bain, since the patient is less than 10 kg. These circuits are lightweight and portable, provide low resistance to respiration, and allow you to control respirations effectively.**

5. Emergence   No special considerations.

6. Intraop problems

a. *Dropping oxygen saturation:* Remember, the brain goes bad before the eyes do. Go to 100% oxygen and hand ventilate while you figure out the problem. Small children have a difference of only a few centimeters between extubation and endobronchial intubation. Especially if the head is moved back and forth and up and down, the endotracheal tube may go awry. Listen to the lungs, feel the bag, suction the ET tube, and if necessary move the surgeons out of the way and take a look with the laryngoscope to make sure you're in the right place.

b. *Bucking on the tube* in spite of neuromuscular relaxation: The diaphragm is hard to block, *especially if the CO_2 is high. Bucking is hypercapnia until proven otherwise.*

POSTOP

1. Apnea   If the child is less than 60 weeks' gestational age, then he will be prone to postoperative apnea. Apnea monitoring for 24 hours postop is mandatory. Even after 60 weeks' gestational age, a premature child may be susceptible to postoperative apnea. Postop apnea monitoring is needed for premature infants for 24 hours. The age at which postop apnea monitoring is no longer needed for a premature child is unclear. Most centers monitor them for 24 hours postop until the child is 1 year old.

2. Stridor   Small children have small, easily obstructed airways. The slightest amount of circumferential edema can dramatically reduce the caliber of the airway. The air flow through the narrowed airway produces sounds of turbulence. Consider other causes such as aspiration of a foreign body. If the stridor is from edema, treat with humidified oxygen and inhaled racemic epinephrine. If the resistance to breathing becomes so great that the child cannot maintain adequate ventilation, reintubation with a smaller tube is the next step.

"Why did they say that! I'd never do it that way!" you say.

That's what we want to hear. Keep banging away at it. Check up on what we said or come up with your own answers.

CASE 9   *(word/phrase approach)*

A 60-year-old, 89 kg male, a former all-star wrestler, is admitted for emergency resection of an abdominal aortic aneurysm (AAA). He has had abdominal pain for the past 4 hours. His last meal was a chile slaw dog washed down with a Lalapalooza milk shake a few hours ago. Meds: Lopressor (metoprolol tartrate) and minoxidil. BP 200/100; P 100; Hct 42.

60 years old, 89 kg
emergency AAA

Pre op — Vitals: ↑ BP   ⟩ ↑ myocard O₂ demand
                    ↑ HR

              Angio : size of aneurysm
                       location of aneurysm

      Labs: ECG , Lytes , CBC w/diff
             PT/PTT

Assume all these patients have significant coronary artery disease. Other notes to put on the page under this stem include:

1. *Renal considerations:*

Bun /cr - pre op

Loc of x clamp - renal compromise.

may need Dopamine
Mannitol

2. Central administration of drugs:

3. Unclamping:

Lopressor and minoxidil   Use the generic names of medications on the exam. You would hate to have the examiner ask you the *real* name of Lopressor and only be able to answer with an embarrassed grin.

What does minoxidil have to do with anesthesia?

As a last resort, you can say that you would take the time to review the drug in Stoelting's *Anesthesia and Co-existing Disease* (the interactions of most commonly used drugs with anesthetic agents can be found there) and the *PDR*.

BP 200/100, P 100   Going to do anything about it?

Hct 42 The classic question on this is, "So the patient hasn't bled, right?"

Now our version.

~~~~~~~~~~~~~~~~~

60 years old, 89 kg Not significant.

emergency AAA Envision a variety of induction scenarios, from a stable patient with plenty of time for line placement to a moribund patient with a rapidly distending abdomen. In the stable patient you want big IV lines, an A-line, and a pulmonary artery catheter. In the moribund patient, you intubate instantly and forge ahead with clamping that aorta.

With any emergency aneurysm, assume a full stomach and, presumably, a bad heart. You don't have time to work the patient up at your leisure. Assume cardiac disease and induce accordingly. Titrate narcotic in before you perform the rapid sequence induction. If the patient has lost lots of blood, even a combination of narcotics and etomidate may be enough to kill him by relaxing his sympathetic tone. Therefore try to check filling pressures before you induce. If the patient is hemodynamically *stable* and hypovolemic, *treat* the hypovolemia before you induce. If you do not have time (the aneurysm has ruptured), then reduce your doses of narcotic and induction agent.

Assume that all these patients have significant coronary artery disease. Other notes to put on the page under this stem include:

1. *Renal considerations:* Preserve renal blood flow and renal tubular flow. Infuse low-dose dopamine and give mannitol one-half hour before the aorta is clamped, if possible.

2. *Central administration of drugs:* Central access for administration of vasoactive drugs is mandatory. Even if the patient is hemodynamically stable, clamping the aorta can induce marked increases in

afterload and left ventricular dysfunction/failure. With the aorta cross-clamped, a CVP catheter does not reliably track left-sided filling pressures. A PA catheter is mandatory. (This statement is controversial.)

3. *Unclamping:* Hydrate to a wedge pressure greater than normal for that patient, or else to 15 to 17 mm Hg. Check blood gases after unclamping to determine the need for bicarbonate administration.

Lopressor and minoxidil   Use the generic names of medications on the exam. You would hate to have the examiner ask you the *real* name of Lopressor and only be able to answer with an embarrassed grin.

What does minoxidil have to do with anesthesia? Will anything weird happen, besides perhaps a little extra hair growth? Sooner or later you will confront a drug whose effects you can't really remember. Go with your gut instinct—if the drug had a specific weird association with anesthesia, you would probably have heard about it by the end of your residency. (Minoxidil, by the by, just causes some fluid retention and reflex tachycardia, no big deal).

As a last resort, you can say that you would take the time to review the drug in Stoelting's *Anesthesia and Co-existing Disease* (the interactions of most commonly used drugs with anesthetic agents can be found there) and the *PDR*.

BP 200/100, P 100   Going to do anything about it? Should you just figure, "Well, pretty soon he'll be asleep so it'll come down then and it'll be gravy"? Think again. If you let the pressure and pulse stay that high for too long, the patient really *will* be asleep—forever! Treat the hypertension and tachycardia now (labetalol hydrochloride would be OK) to prevent dangerous stress on the aneurysm.

Hct 42   The classic question on this is, "So the patient hasn't bled, right?" Wrong. The hematocrit does not drop commensurate with bleeding. Equilibration (extravascular fluid diluting down remaining blood cells) following hemorrhage takes hours, unless the patient has been rigorously volume repleted. A "normal" hematocrit does not necessarily mean that the patient has not bled.

CASE 10   *(preop/intraop/postop approach)*

A 54-year-old, 95 kg male with acute cholecystitis is admitted for emergency cholecystectomy. He had a gastric resection 5 years ago, and has required 4 days of respiratory care due to asthma. The pa-

tient frequently uses bronchodilators, especially in cold weather.
BP 170/90; P 80; R 14; WBC 15,000; Hgb 16; T 39°C.

Last time you get any clues at all.

PREOP

1. Labs PFTs to the tune of $FEV_1/FRC \downarrow$, $FRC \uparrow$, $FEV_1 \downarrow$

$MMEF_{25-75}$ – small

2. Consults The best consult would be the old chart,

If the case were elective, a pulmonary consult to optimize bronchodilator therapy for 48–72 hrs prior to Sx.

3. Further medical therapy Examine the chest to see if the patient is Actively wheezing

1. Special considerations

Full stomach: Can you have a full stomach when you don't have a stomach?

yes

How about drugs like cimetidine or metoclopramide in this agastric patient?

No use

Postop ventilation:

2. Monitors   A-line

monitor Bl gases

3. Induction   Full stomach and bronchospastic disease puts you in double jeopardy:

Rapid sequence

4. Maintenance   Enflurane or isoflurane/oxygen/relaxant. All inhaled agents

5. Emergence   Although a deep extubation would prevent the patient from reacting to the endotracheal tube, deep extubation is unacceptable for two reasons:

    1.   Full stomach

    2.

Since he required such long postop ventilation last time,

6. Intraop problems

    a. *Bronchospasm:* All that wheezes is not asthma.

In the nth degree of bronchospasm, after all else has failed and *only* after all else has failed (i.e., the patient is going to die),

b. *Biliary spasm on the cholangiogram:*

POSTOP

1. Agitation   Agitation is always, *always* _____ until proven otherwise:

2. Bronchospasm   You hit a kind of catch-22 here. Extubating the patient may relieve the stimulus causing bronchospasm, but

The search for other causes of bronchospasm should continue in the postoperative period:

Read 'em and weep.

~~~~~~~~~~~~~~~~

PREOP

1. Labs PFTs to the tune of FEV_1, FVC, $MMEF_{25-75}$, and $PEFR_{200-1200}$ with and without bronchodilators would be optimal. Because of the acute nature of the illness, that may not be possible.

Room air blood gases. Given the patient's earlier respiratory troubles, you will need baseline blood gases to guide postoperative weaning.

Theophylline level—yes and no. If he is actually taking Theo-Dur now, you will want to establish the blood level so you don't overdose him. If, of course, he is not presently taking theophylline, a blood level is meaningless.

2. Consults The best consult would be the old chart, detailing the specific cause and course of the patient's postop ventilation.

If the procedure were elective, a pulmonary consult to optimize bronchodilator therapy for 48 to 72 hours preoperatively would decrease the risk of postoperative pulmonary complications.

3. Further medical therapy Examine the chest to see if the patient is wheezing. Give an inhaled beta agent prior to induction. If he is wheezing, load with aminophylline. The case is not so urgent that you must begin before starting therapy for bronchospastic disease.

INTRAOP

1. Special considerations

Full stomach: Can you have a full stomach when you don't have a stomach? (Recall that the patient had a gastric resection.) Well, yes, we would consider this emergency patient who has a process interfering with normal peristalsis as having a full stomach. It might be more accurate to say, full upper intestinal tract. How about drugs like cimetidine or metoclopramide in this agastric patient? We would say no, because the increased contractility caused by metoclopramide may work for you or against you—it depends on what is hooked to what in the intestinal tract. The H_2 blockers would not help either—the parietal cells of the stomach are in some pathology jar somewhere!

Postop ventilation: Assuming that the problem was asthma/bronchospasm, the use of bronchodilators and bronchodilating anesthetics would be appropriate.

2. Monitors   A-line for frequent blood gases. Consider a pulmonary artery catheter. This man may not need it for the operation, but he will need delicate postop fluid management if his lungs are ever to get optimized enough so that he can be extubated.

3. Induction   Full stomach and bronchospastic disease puts you in double jeopardy. The high white cell count, fever, and the word from the surgeons (if they feel it is emergent, well then, it is) all rob you of the luxury of breathing the patient deep before instrumenting the airway. (Some would argue for relaxant and pentothal, followed by O_2 plus inhalation agent by mask with cricoid pressure.) Even though you haven't got all the time in the world to blunt the patient's response to intubation, you can lower it somewhat. Titrate in some narcotic before beginning a rapid sequence induction. If he has no cardiac disease, then ketamine (preceded by an anticholinergic to control secretions) is the agent of choice for a rapid sequence induction. If he has cardiac disease, then use relatively large doses of etomidate or pentothal if ventricular function is good. The utility of lidocaine in blunting the response to intubation is controversial. We would give it. Your goal here is to secure the airway quickly without precipitating bronchospasm, no mean feat.

4. Maintenance   Enflurane or isoflurane/oxygen/relaxant. All inhaled agents have the same amount of bronchodilation. Using halothane while running in aminophylline increases the risk of ventricular arrhythmias. Because of the history of asthma during the patient's last perioperative course, attempt to maximize the amount of bronchodilation by using pure inhalation technique. Use pancuronium for relaxation. It is a sympathomimetic and will help with bronchodilation. If your other bronchodilator therapy has already induced an unacceptable tachycardia, give vecuronium.

5. Emergence Although a deep extubation would prevent the patient from reacting to the endotracheal tube, deep extubation is unacceptable for two reasons:

1. Full stomach at induction: aspiration is possible
2. Postop ventilation may be necessary

Since he required such long postop ventilation last time, a low threshold for keeping him intubated is appropriate. Better to keep him intubated a little longer than to have to reintubate.

6. Intraop problems

a. *Bronchospasm:* All that wheezes is not asthma. Pneumothorax, aspiration, endobronchial intubation, ET tube against the carina, kinks in the tube, and mucous plugs in the ET tube or airways can all increase airway pressures and cause audible turbulent flow. Rule these out by listening to both sides of the chest, passing a suction catheter, and adjusting the position of the ET tube. Once you have ruled out *other* causes of wheezing, then treat bronchospasm. Deepen the level of anesthesia with oxygen and enflurane or isoflurane. If this is not successful, try beta inhalers, aminophylline, steroids (if you are anticipating a long bout with bronchospasm), and maybe even an epinephrine drip if your back is to the wall.

In the nth degree of bronchospasm, after all else has failed and *only* after all else has failed (i.e., the patient is going to die), pull out the ET tube and mask the patient. This is obviously a last-ditch approach.

b. *Biliary spasm on the cholangiogram:* Narcotics may have precipitated this. Treatment with naloxone is effective but undoes your analgesia. Nitroglycerin works, as does glucagon (usual glucagon dose, 1 mg).

POSTOP

1. Agitation Agitation is always, *always* hypoxemia until proven otherwise. Check blood gases, hand ventilate the patient if he is intubated, give ventilatory assist by mask if he is not. Only after you have *proven adequacy of ventilation* should you turn to other causes of agitation: hypo- or hyperglycemia, hyponatremia, anticholinergic effects, pain, distended bladder or stomach. A full differential of postoperative delirium is discussed in Case 7. In approaching this problem remember to organize your response by subdividing potential causes into drug-related, metabolic, and neurologic categories. A head-to-toe search for a cause of agitation should precede any sedative or pain relief.

2. Bronchospasm You hit a kind of catch-22 here. Extubating the patient may relieve the stimulus causing bronchospasm, but he may need prolonged ventilatory support. Prudence dictates continuing to maximize therapy until the bronchospasm is under control, rather than extubating right away.

The search for other causes of bronchospasm should continue in the postoperative period. Pneumothorax, malposition of the ET tube, and other mishaps can still occur.

CASE 11 *(word/phrase approach)*

An 82-year-old, 65 kg male is admitted for bronchoscopy and right upper lobe resection for epidermoid carcinoma of the lung. The patient was a heavy cigarette smoker and has a chronic cough. He has had hypertension for 10 years. The ECG shows Q waves in the inferior leads. BP 170/90; P 84; T 38°C; Hgb 11.

Almost on your own.

82 years old

65 kg plus lung cancer

heavy smoker with chronic cough

Preparing for the Anesthesia Orals

thoracotomy

Sample Questions

mild hypertension with BP 170/90

Preparing for the Anesthesia Orals

Q waves in the inferior leads

Here's what we thought.

Sample Questions

82 years old All the considerations for the elderly. Decreased reserve in all organ systems. He needs light or no premedication since respiratory depression in the sick elderly patient can occur at drug dosages that would not normally cause any respiratory problems in younger patients.

65 kg plus lung cancer Malnutrition from chronic disease or metastases. Check this before surgery and consider nutritional support preoperatively if there is severe malnutrition. Preoperative nutritional support has been associated with a decreased incidence of postoperative complications and enhanced wound healing. The patient probably has a low albumin level and thus higher bioavailability of protein-bound drugs. Consider a possible myasthenic response to neuromuscular blockers (Eaton-Lambert syndrome).

heavy smoker with chronic cough How do you know when this patient will be optimized? You want to clear up any infection preop (get a chest x-ray), but his infection may be impossible to eradicate (socked-in pneumonia behind an obstructing carcinoma). PFTs? Once again, FVC, FEV_1, $MMEF_{25-75}$ both before and after bronchodilators. Also, a room air arterial blood gas. (This exact battery of pulmonary function tests should sound familiar.) If there is evidence of improvement in lung function after bronchodilator therapy, the case must be postponed. As we stated before, 48 to 72 hours of therapy associated with an improvement in PFTs will lessen the incidence of postoperative pulmonary complications.

thoracotomy Routine monitoring here includes an arterial catheter for checking blood gases. An increased alveolar to arterial oxygen gradient is associated with minimal changes in arterial saturation. This is due to the shape of the oxygen-hemoglobin dissociation curve. There may be widened (amount unknown) arterial to end-tidal CO_2 gradient with one-lung ventilation due to V/Q mismatch. These two facts mean that a pulse oximeter and end-tidal CO_2 monitor alone without an A-line are *not* adequate for this case. Be ready to draw why the arterial–end-tidal CO_2 gradient increases with either shunt or dead space (Figure 4). You must be prepared for a pneumonectomy. If the lung function studies indicate that the patient may be a pulmonary cripple after a pneumonectomy, then split lung function studies must be done before the operation. The examiners will try to get you to back down by having an argumentative surgeon give reason after reason why this case must be done immediately (patient convenience, the uncorrectable

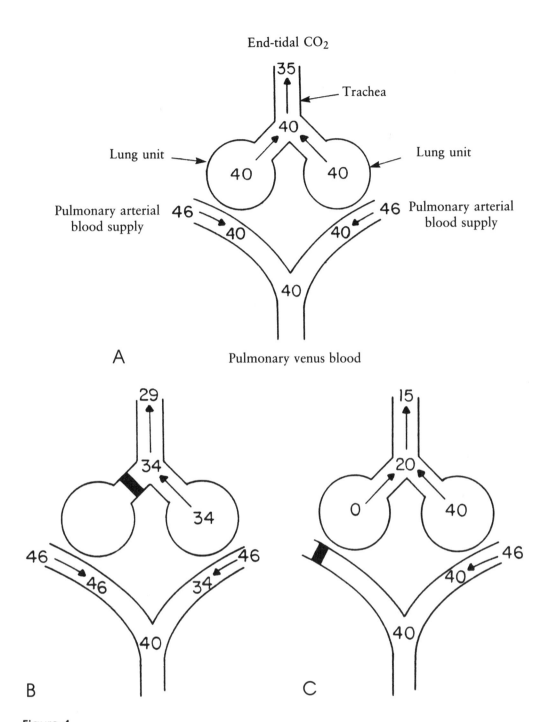

Figure 4
These highly simplified diagrams show why the end-tidal to arterial CO_2 gradient increases with either shunt or dead space. The numbers represent pCO_2 values in mmHg. (A) Normal. Note that the end-tidal CO_2 is 35 rather than 40 because the trachea "dilutes" the alveolar air with CO_2-free air. (B) Shunt. If an arterial pCO_2 of 40 is maintained, then more CO_2 must be unloaded in the section of the lung that is not blocked off. As a result, the end-tidal to arterial CO_2 gradient increases. (C) Dead space. The area of lung that has no blood supply "dilutes" the end-tidal CO_2. As a result, the end-tidal CO_2 gradient increases. Keep in mind that these diagrams are highly simplified. A "pure" shunt or "pure" dead space, devoid of patient response (vasoconstriction, rerouting blood flow, and ventilation), does not exist.

pneumonia, "I'm only going to take out a lobe, don't be ridiculous"). Stand your ground.

A double-lumen tube may be mandatory. If there is a right-sided pulmonary infection and the surgeons think their manipulation may expose the opposite lung to purulent contamination, then the double-lumen tube must be placed and the bronchial cuff inflated during the entire procedure. If not, the double-lumen tube is optional.

The intraoperative complications you can expect have been discussed in other questions. Our repetition is purposeful. Hypoxia is guaranteed. A quick evaluation that you are indeed delivering 100% oxygen to the good lung should be followed by applying CPAP to the deflated lung, PEEP to the inflated lung, then differential CPAP/PEEP to both lungs. Ventilating the deflated lung is a surgical inconvenience but may be a life-saving action on your part. All vasodilators reduce hypoxic pulmonary vasoconstriction, as does greater than 1 MAC of inhaled agents.

mild hypertension with BP 170/90 You will be asked if you will cancel the case. If you believe what we wrote earlier, you won't cancel, since the diastolic pressure is not above 110 mm Hg. Look for any associated end-organ damage that may have resulted from the hypertension (renal insufficiency, heart failure, stroke, angina). If these are present, it would be prudent to treat the blood pressure before bringing the patient to the OR. Don't let the blood pressure drop too low. (Exact recommendations are exceedingly difficult to make.) As an empirical rule, keep the blood pressure no lower than 30% below the patient's normal mean arterial blood pressure. Theoretically that should keep the blood pressure in the range where cerebral autoregulation provides constant cerebral blood flow. Cerebral autoregulation is shifted to the right in the chronically hypertensive patient (although when they ask you how far it is shifted and how long blood pressure has to be treated before cerebral autoregulation shifts to the left, you may be forced to throw up your arms, plead ignorance, and beg for mercy). Coronary perfusion pressure will probably remain adequate as well, if the blood pressure is kept near normal.

Q waves in the inferior leads This is a real pain. Your main job is to use old charts and the history to find out when the myocardial infarction occurred (the patient may not have a clue), compare the ECG to an old one to see if *you* can figure out when it happened (during your exam, there won't be an old ECG available), and figure out how impaired the ventricle is. If you really can't determine whether some of the patient's shortness of breath is cardiac in origin, you might have to ask Cardiology for an echocardiogram or MUGA scan. If the echocardiogram or MUGA scan shows poor ventricular function, then you may need a pulmonary artery catheter to monitor volume status intraoperatively. Poor LV function will also push you away from potent inhaled agents and toward a more narcotic-based technique.

A technique geared toward a poor myocardium is more likely to result in postoperative ventilatory support. Although such ventilatory support exposes a fresh bronchial stump to positive pressure, we would still use narcotics if there were left ventricular dysfunction: better to get the patient through the operation stable and on a ventilator than to push for early extubation. (You can choose the opposite approach and still satisfy the examiners' need to evaluate your judgment and clarity of presentation. "Even with ventricular dysfunction, I would titrate in an inhaled agent while following left ventricular performance—cardiac output versus preload. This would enhance the likelihood of early extubation and decrease the possibility of positive-pressure ventilation ripping the suture line on the bronchial stump.)

By now you should be gaining a bit of confidence in your ability to analyze a stem question.

CASE 12 *(preop/intraop/postop approach)*

A 66-year-old, 62 kg female with a 30-year history of rheumatoid arthritis is admitted for a total hip replacement. Rx: 60 mg prednisone daily along with acetylsalicylic acid as needed. Glucose 135; Hct 35; BP 140/80; P 80; R 14.

PREOP

  1. Labs

2. Consults

3. Further medical therapy

INTRAOP

    1. Special considerations

    2. Monitors

Sample Questions

3. Induction

4. Maintenance

5. Emergence

6. Intraop problems

Preparing for the Anesthesia Orals

1. **Addisonian crisis**

2. **Pulmonary embolus**

3. **ARDS**

Our plan.

~~~~~~~~~~~~~~~~~~~

PREOP

1. **Labs**   Rheumatoid arthritis (RA) affects the body systemically, so a head-to-toe search for pathology is indicated.

C-spine x-ray: Yes, you could order one because these patients can have atlanto-occipital subluxation. If the patient has no symptoms even on neck extension, we would not order one. If you do get the x-ray and it shows cervical pathology, you must be extra careful when extending the neck. Consider an awake fiberoptic intubation.

Sample Questions

Chest x-ray: Rheumatoid lung can be anything from nodules to almost an ARDS picture. Check the chest x-ray for any such signs.

BUN and creatinine: A systemic vasculitis accompanies RA. The kidneys may be involved.

ECG and old ECG: The patient's age and the possibility of associated conduction defects in RA make this a necessity.

Physical exam: Every patient needs a physical exam, of course, but the airway exam requires meticulous attention in patients with RA. Every facet of the airway, from the C-spine to TMJ to the arytenoids, can be anatomically abnormal and present obstructions to intubation.

Bleeding time: Another maybe. In general, most patients coming to the OR who are on aspirin do not need a bleeding time. Since a lot of blood loss may be involved in this case, we would get a bleeding time if the patient were taking lots of aspirin.

2. Consults   If you *do* order a cervical film, you might as well ask a radiologist for an official reading. If there is atlanto-occipital subluxation, the opinion of a neurosurgeon is warranted. In any case, be sure to say that you will be careful when manipulating the neck.

3. Further medical therapy   None needed.

INTRAOP

1. Special considerations   The hematocrit of 35 is suspicious in a little old lady with a broken hip and longstanding disease. Most likely she is dehydrated, and the hematocrit of 35 represents hemoconcentration rather than robust health.

Airway, airway, airway. If in doubt, always take an awake look.

The lateral position is often uncomfortable and can make a regional technique problematic. If you use a regional and the patient needs a general anesthetic later on, you'll have to ask the surgeons to stop and turn the patient supine.

You can bet that the examiners will be testing your adaptability during this case. First, they will make securing the airway a problem. Be prepared and have a first, second, and third plan (awake look, nasal fiberoptic, cricothyrotomy/trach). Can you avoid intubating the patient and really do the hip under regional for the exam? It is very doubtful that the examiners will let you get away with this. They will have the regional technique fail or make up a complication like an intravascular injection followed by a seizure and the need to protect the airway. Then you'll be doing an impossible intubation emergently.

What a blast! If you anticipate how the examiners may manipulate the case, you won't be flustered and you'll pass. Simple as that.

2. Monitors   A-line for frequent hematocrits, Foley catheter, and CVP line. Hip surgery is associated with large fluid shifts (from the patient to the floor), and little old ladies with fractured hips are invariably as dry as bone to begin with. Plunk in that CVP line and *treat hypovolemia* before you induce.

3. Induction   If the airway is a real problem, tackle it head on. Intubate awake with a topical and sedation. If you try to tiptoe around the airway with a regional technique, that technique will fail for sure. This dictum of oral boards was stated before, but it bears repeating.

If the airway is not a problem and the patient has the mental facility to hold still for a regional technique, then a spinal or epidural would be fine after adequate fluid loading. A slick way to handle the spinal is to position the patient with her bad hip up and in a slight Trendelenburg position, put the needle subarachnoid, inject a dose of a hypobaric long-acting local anesthetic, then keep the needle in. If the level is inadequate, inject some more local anesthetic.

4. Maintenance   Whatever.

5. Emergence   If the airway was difficult to secure, extubate only when the patient is fully awake.

6. Intraop problems

a. *Inability to intubate,* even when the patient is awake. If you can't intubate with a fiberoptic scope or by awake looks with the laryngoscope, you will need progressively more exotic techniques. You can try a retrograde wire up the trachea. That is done so rarely that few practitioners have the requisite skill. Don't suggest it unless you can do it—the examiners will not be fooled or amused. Every now and then a plain old blind nasal will drop the endotracheal tube in.

When you're stuck, you're stuck. If trach you must, then so be it.

b. *Agitation* halfway through the case with the patient under spinal. Before you reach for the sedative, *check your pulse oximeter and blood gases!* Old people with possibly altered mentation can aspirate; emboli from the artificial hip area can adversely affect oxygenation (by liquefied fat or glue globs or some weird thing); and any number of other sinister things could happen. Don't just sedate for agitation.

POSTOP

1. Addisonian crisis   Come on, do you really think that if you don't replace the steroids, your patient will have an addisonian crisis? In our heart of hearts we just don't know if we believe that. For your board of boards, believe it.

2. Pulmonary embolus   Suddenly the patient becomes dyspneic, agitated, and perhaps cyanotic. Start supplemental oxygen, and secure the airway if supplemental oxygen does not improve the saturation. Start fluids and pressors, if necessary, to support circulation. Depending on the degree of circulatory compromise, the patient may require a pulmonary artery catheter.

Why should this patient have a pulmonary embolism? Old, debilitated, immobile, orthopedic long bone injury—a classic setup for thromboemboli or fat emboli.

3. ARDS   If the patient has had a fat embolus, ARDS will inevitably follow (at least on the exam)—you can't do anything about it. Give PEEP only when the patient needs it and keep the preload adequate for oxygen delivery. Expect and treat concomitant infections.

By now you should be able to invent likely complications and lines of reasoning that the examiners will follow.

CASE 13   *(word/phrase approach)*

A 28-year-old, 55 kg female, G9P8, widow (her husband died of exhaustion 3 weeks earlier), pregnant (36 weeks' gestation), presents with brisk vaginal bleeding and crampy pelvic pain. BP 80/60; P 130; R 20; FHR 180.

vaginal bleeding and pelvic pain

Preparing for the Anesthesia Orals

BP 80/60, P 130

Sample Questions

FHR 180

Preparing for the Anesthesia Orals

vaginal bleeding and pelvic pain Placenta previa and placental abruption are at the top of the differential. Place some large-bore IV lines and send blood for a quick type and screen, hematocrit, platelets, PT, PTT, fibrin split products, fibrinogen. Disseminated intravascular coagulation is a possibility that must be addressed. Regional technique? Negative: cut off sympathetic tone in a patient already bleeding and you court disaster.

Ultrasound is the best way of getting a quick diagnosis. A digital exam is only allowable once the IV lines have been placed, blood is available, and the patient is in the OR prepped and draped for immediate C-section.

BP 80/60, P 130 Don't forget *left uterine displacement!* Tachycardia and hypotension equal hypovolemia. Without left uterine displacement, hypovolemia is exacerbated. Gear your induction to the hypovolemic state, i.e., use ketamine. But keep in mind that even ketamine may act as a myocardial depressant if the patient is maxed out on her stress response. Also beware uterine hypertonus with a dose of ketamine greater than 1 mg/kg, especially given a hypertonic uterus to start with in placental abruption. Give colloid since it will replete the intravascular volume faster than cystalloid, and time is of the essence. Do it before you start the induction, if at all possible. Volume, volume, volume.

If the blood pressure goes down any more, *your first responsibility is to the mother.* Be prepared to act decisively in favor of the mother. Phenylephrine and epinephrine should be given to prevent damage to her vital organs, i.e., if the mean blood pressure is below 50. These pressors have a short half-life, and when volume resuscitation is better you can revert to ephedrine. With the mother already pouring out catecholamines, the indirect-acting ephedrine is useless in a crisis.

A coding mother may mean emergency delivery if the fetus is compromised. The infant will have a better chance, and the chest compressions will be more effective for the mother.

FHR 180 The rate of 180 is above the upper limits of normal, indicating fetal stress (persistent fetal tachycardia). The most likely cause of stress is the mother's hypovolemia. Giving supplemental oxygen to the mother is a benign and mandatory maneuver. Continue volume resuscitating and make sure you have good left uterine displacement.

Sample Questions

For any OB question, the examiners will ask you about fetal heart rates and patterns. In brief:

Variable decelerations are usually not sinister unless frequent and
  severe
Late decelerations are a sign of distress
Early decelerations are a sign of head compression
Decelerations below 60 or a deceleration for > 60 seconds equals
  serious distress
Loss of variability occurs with stress, neurologic injury, or under
  general anesthesia, or with the epidural administration of local
  anesthetics.

Given the patient's state and the sign of fetal distress, prepare for emergency C-section. Make sure the patient has had a nonparticulate antacid before coming to the OR.

Do you get a fetal scalp pH for further assessment? Of course not. The placenta may be overlying the cervical os, so an attempt at measuring fetal scalp pH could exacerbate the hemorrhage. If this were a straightforward question of fetal distress, you would go to C-section if the fetal scalp pH were less than 7.20.

If you are delivering a distressed baby, be ready to resuscitate. If the Apgar is less than 3, you have no time to lose. Immediate intubation and 100% oxygen by positive-pressure ventilation is usually sufficient. If not, administration of epinephrine and atropine down the endotracheal tube is the next step while you call for help and get an umbilical artery catheter placed. Once again, if the infant and mother both need resuscitation simultaneously, you must not direct attention to the infant until the mother's resuscitation is being managed by another qualified physician or until the mother's resuscitation is successful.

CASE 14   *(preop/intraop/postop approach)*

A 60-year-old, 70 kg male is admitted for right carotid endarterectomy. He has a history of episodes of transient ischemic attacks (TIAs) and longstanding hypertension. Rx: hydralazine, furosemide, propranolol. BP 190/110; P 60; R 18; ECG shows sinus bradycardia and left anterior hemiblock.

Preparing for the Anesthesia Orals

PREOP

1. Labs   *EKg –*

2. Consults

cardiac

3. Further medical therapy

133   *Sample Questions*

INTRAOP

    1. Special considerations

    2. Monitors

Preparing for the Anesthesia Orals

3. Induction

4. Maintenance

Sample Questions

5. Emergence

6. Intraop problems

POSTOP
1. Hematoma

2. Chest pain

3. Stroke

Preparing for the Anesthesia Orals

4. Delayed awakening

Our answer.

~~~~~~~~~~~~~~~~~~~~

1. Labs   Hypertension mandates a look for end-organ damage, so check BUN and creatinine. Furosemide wastes potassium, so check that. Old ECG to compare (always).

2. Consults   You should be able to answer questions pertaining to angina and left ventricular function after a history and physical exam. The hard question is, "Does this patient have myocardium at risk for ischemia?" That question may best be answered by a dipyridamole-thallium perfusion scan.

One question for the cardiologists is, "With this patient's sinus bradycardia and left anterior hemiblock, are we sure the TIAs are TIAs or are we having syncope of cardiac origin?" A Holter monitor may answer that question. You would hate to have the patient undergo an unnecessary procedure. In the exam, this would best be phrased "Assuming that a cardiac origin for the syncopal episodes had been ruled out. . . ."

3. Further medical therapy   The blood pressure is a tad high. Postpone the case until the blood pressure is under better control. Post carotid endarterectomy hypertension is most frequently associated with preoperative hypertension. Sustained systolic hypertension (>200 mm Hg) is associated with increased postoperative neurologic morbidity after carotid surgery. Furthermore, a diastolic of 110 mm Hg is a cutoff for cancelling elective cases. Such a high blood pressure is associated with greater incidence of postoperative cardiopulmonary complications.

The examiners will try to make you change your mind about canceling the case by saying that the patient could stroke out because you delayed. Respond, "The patient is more likely to have a negative outcome from his poor medical condition than from delaying the case." The examiners may then throw you another curve ball and say, "The patient is having frequent and current ongoing TIAs." You may then have to *adapt* (grading criteria, remember?) to the patient's changed clinical condition and to the operation under suboptimal conditions, *judging* that the risk of thrombotic stroke is greater than a complication secondary to hypertension.

INTRAOP

1. Special considerations   After an actual stroke, wait at least 4 to 6 weeks before performing an elective operation. Perioperative mortality is sky-high in the patient with such a recent stroke. TIAs do not count as strokes.

The risk of coronary artery disease is very high. Even with a negative history and no need for a further workup, cardiac dysfunction/ischemia should be high on your differential if the patient decompensates.

The patient must be arousable immediately postoperatively so that neurologic function can be assessed.

2. Monitors   Whether regional or general anesthesia is used, an arterial line is mandatory for following beat-to-beat blood pressure. Maintaining adequate cerebral perfusion is key to this case. The examiners have been known to ask, "Can't you just use an automated blood pressure cuff in the stat mode?" If you answer no, what then will you say to the examiners' "why?" The rapid swings in blood pressure seen with carotid artery and carotid sinus manipulation make a q30 second pressure inadequate. The machine will cycle only within a certain range of the last blood pressure and will recycle if it takes more than 30 seconds to register a pressure. Several cycles (minutes) may go by if the blood pressure changes are dramatic. Since the blood pressure must be monitored closely throughout the entire case, the continual stat mode would lead to arm ischemia.

Neurologic status monitoring, especially around carotid clamp time, is now routine unless a shunt is placed bypassing the carotid clamps. Monitoring may be done awake with grip strength and with counting. With general anesthesia, slowing and decreased amplitude on EEG or a processed EEG signal (CSA, compressed spectral analysis) is used to diagnose cerebral ischemia.

3. Induction   Regional deep cervical plexus block or general anesthesia may be employed. Regional anesthesia has the advantage of allowing ongoing monitoring by letting you talk with the patient, and hypotension is unusual. Regional anesthesia can be disadvantageous if the patient becomes agitated and you have to induce general anesthesia and control the airway with the patient partially draped and with an open neck wound. Intubating a patient under such conditions is less than ideal.

General anesthesia provides you with airway control but you lose the ability to monitor the patient by talking to him. Induction usually involves some narcotic to blunt the hemodynamic response to intubation (not a high dose, though, since you must wake the patient immediately after the operation to assess neuro status), some pentothal, and some isoflurane, and away you go. Granted, it's the usual garbage anesthetic. The goal on induction is to prevent wide swings in hemodynamics. Hypotension is treated aggressively to prevent inadequate cerebral perfusion.

4. Maintenance   High-dose narcotics are an unsatisfactory option. Isoflurane/nitrous/oxygen will bear the brunt of the anesthetic duty. Does isoflurane afford more protection than the other inhaled agents? Theoretically, yes. Isoflurane provides the most favorable cerebral metabolic rate/cerebral blood flow ratio and may be associated with fewer postoperative neurologic complications.

CO_2: high, low, or normal? Robin Hood, anti-Robin Hood, the Sheriff of Nottingham and good King Richard. It's like a fairy tale, not much real evidence. The current recommendation is to keep the CO_2 normal or slightly low in order to prevent cerebral steal.

The examiners may push you to explain steal in either the coronary or cerebral circulation. The theory is as follows: There are areas of tissue downstream from a vascular obstruction that are at risk of ischemia if the blood flow is at all decreased. The vasculature in these "at risk" areas is already maximally dilated. If you dilate (with CO_2 in this case) vascular beds in "not at risk" tissue, then a larger portion of the fixed blood flow will be distributed away from the "at risk" tissue.

5. Emergence   The patient must be aroused from slumber quickly so you can do a neuro check. Due to the possibility of coexisting cardiac disease, you don't want emergence accompanied by hypertension and tachycardia. Treat such aberrations quickly with, for example, labetolol.

A stormy emergence with violent bucking may place a lot of stress on the fresh neck wound. A large hematoma there could lead to airway compromise. The carotid sutures themselves may pop off if the patient strains too much. Given these caveats, smooth the emergence by judicious narcotic or lidocaine administration.

6. Intraop problems

a. *Nausea during a regional block:* Think hypotension. Any number of odd hemodynamic changes can happen during carotid manipulation. These can lead to hypotension, and the awake patient becomes nauseated. Intraoperative hemodynamic changes include bradycardia and hypotension from carotid sinus manipulation, and hypertension with carotid sheath/artery manipulation. Hypotension and bradycardia can follow reperfusion of the carotid. The transmission of a relatively bounding pulse through the newly stripped intima makes the carotid sinus believe that the blood pressure is high when it is really normal. The baroreceptors then respond by producing hypotension and bradycardia.

What can you do? Have the surgeons instill lidocaine at the carotid sinus to blunt its overreactive response. Hypotension and bradycardia unresponsive to this maneuver should immediately be treated with neosynephrine, fluids, and atropine.

b. *EEG changes consistent with ischemia:* Something has altered cerebral perfusion and you must fix it pronto. The most common cause is an embolus (the horse is out of the barn there, not much you can do about an embolus). If ischemic changes occur at the time of carotid artery clamping, placement of a shunt and/or removal of the clamp is mandatory. Other causes include hypotension (the mean blood pressure should optimally be maintained at 20% above the resting mean arterial pressure) and head position (a sharply turned neck may cut off blood supply).

Preparing for the Anesthesia Orals

POSTOP

1. Hematoma A rapidly expanding hematoma can cause airway compromise. In such a case you face the dilemma, "Do I reintubate or do I open the neck?" Reintubate if you can, the patient will be going back to the OR soon. If you cannot pass the ET tube, open the neck. That will relieve the airway compression and facilitate intubation. If the surgeon is not available to open the neck, do it yourself, intubate, and then manually compress the site. He who hesitates is lost.

2. Chest pain Post-carotid endarterectomy patients are at high risk for cardiac events. This episode of chest pain requires the usual treatment: oxygen, morphine, sublingual or IV nitrates, and correction of any factors that place stress on the heart (tachycardia, hypertension). Difficulty treating the chest pain or ECG changes require the patient to go to an ICU to have an MI ruled out. Calcium channel blockers may also help.

3. Stroke If a new neurologic deficit is present postoperatively, the only real treatment is supportive. A quick discussion with the surgeons will reveal whether reexploration will benefit the patient. A complete hemiplegia may be due to carotid artery thrombosis or compression by hematoma. Maintaining an adequate blood pressure may yield some benefit, although if the stroke is embolic in origin, most likely nothing will help.

4. Delayed awakening Postoperative delayed awakening or postoperative delirium is a common question on all exams, especially with neurologic and carotid artery procedures. The examiners' approach to this is often as follows: Typically, a nurse will call you with a complaint that the patient is restless, can she give morphine? Or the nurse says the patient is somnolent, can she give some narcan? If you want to get in trouble, just say yes. Instead, you respond that you will go to the bedside, evaluate life-threatening causes immediately, and check ABC. (Almost every question we've discussed has some problem that requires a quick evaluation of airway, oxygenation, breathing, and hemodynamic stability. That's no coincidence.)

A diagnosis is made by going through your organized differential (drugs, metabolic, and neurologic). Then the *cause* of the altered mental status is treated.

Check ABC—always, for all aberrations, for all patients, all the time, rain or shine.

CASE 15 *(word/phrase approach)*

A 65-year-old, 46 kg woman requires open reduction of a compound fracture of the humerus. The patient fell 4 hours ago. She is lethargic and hoarse. The only medication is thyroid replacement. BP 90/50; P 50; R 10; Hct 30; T 35.6°C.

65 years old

46 kg

compound fracture of humerus

fell 4 hours ago and now lethargic

hoarse and on thyroid replacement

low BP, slow heart rate, low temp

temp 35.6°C

Preparing for the Anesthesia Orals

Hct 30

~~~~~~~~~~~~~~~~~~~~

65 years old   Not ancient, but definitely has decreased reserve function in all organ systems.

46 kg   Small person. Reduce dosages appropriately or you'll be waking her up tomorrow.

compound fracture of humerus   Lot of blood in those fractures. Also, document any neurologic deficit before you start the case. You don't want Joe Lawyer blaming your positioning or the surgery for a nerve injury that was already present preoperatively.

fell 4 hours ago and now lethargic   Associated injuries, associated injuries, a thousand times associated injuries! Check arterial blood gases and glucose, and give supplemental oxygen. Make sure a workup for intracranial bleeding was done if there was any suggestion of associated head trauma. Could the patient have suffered a cervical spine injury? Could she have fractured a rib and be at risk for a tension pneumothorax with positive-pressure ventilation? Why did she fall? Could this have been syncope rather than a simple slip?

Again, controlling the exam, you could preface your therapeutic decisions with the statements, "Assuming that this was straightforward trauma [optional: with no suggestion of a syncopal episode], I would direct my attention to the patient's volume status and possible associated injuries." Don't mention syncope if you can't answer the examiner's question, "OK, she's 'fallen out' a few times before. What would you do differently?" A few things to consider when evaluating a patient with a history of syncope are to get a thorough history concentrating on cardiac and neurologic disease, compare old and new ECGs looking for conduction defects, and get a Holter recording to look for arrhythmias, plus cardiology and neurology consults if time permits.

Always exclude from your answer areas in which you are weak. Don't volunteer to hang yourself.

hoarse and on thyroid replacement DANGER DANGER WILL ROBINSON! This patient may have a difficult airway from soft tissue injury or she may be hypothyroid. The two are not mutually exclusive, she may have both. Plan an awake or fiberoptic look at the larynx. Again, caution on your part is a green light for the examiners to give you a passing mark.

low BP, slow heart rate, low temp Looks like hypothyroidism, smells like hypothyroidism, tastes like hypothyroidism. (You should suspect hypovolemia is contributing to the hypotension.) All the signs of hypothyroidism are there. Everything is slowed down in hypothyroid patients: respiration, heart rate, blood pressure, temperature—everything. Although they don't actually have a decreased MAC, they are very sensitive to the *circulatory* depressant effects of inhaled agents. Ketamine is the induction agent of choice. If you say, "Oh, I'd give a little fentanyl, then I'd give some pentothal, then later I would turn on a little enflurane" (as you always do for every case on earth), you will win a free trip back to the boards next year.

Should you replace her thyroid hormone emergently? Only if there is an emergency—like refractory hypotension and bradycardia. Giving T_3 IV is dangerous (for example, it can cause hypertension and tachyarrhythmias) and can precipitate an addisonian crisis if steroids are not given concomitantly.

Expect postoperative lethargy/delayed emergence. Remember to check ABC and consider other causes (*drugs, metabolic, neurologic*). Don't just assume that a hypothyroid patient's lethargy is due to her hypothyroidism.

temp 35.6°C Expect difficulty maintaining temperature. Anticipate decreased clearance of drugs, especially neuromuscular blockers, decreased MAC, possible coagulopathy, and cardiac arrhythmias with temperatures of 30 to 32°C.

Hct 30 This patient will doubtless have a much lower hematocrit once she is rehydrated. Don't be fooled by the borderline-OK number on admission. Recheck that hematocrit, and pick a value below which you'll transfuse. This patient has no apparent cardiopulmonary problems that would decrease oxygen delivery. Therefore, you do not have to transfuse to a hematocrit of 30, but it is a safe and defendable number.

CASE 16 *(preop/intraop/postop approach)*

A 79-year-old, 70 kg man with a permanent transvenous pacemaker is admitted for elective transurethral resection of the prostate (TURP). BP 140/90; P 64; R 16; Hgb 14.

PREOP

    1. Labs   CBC w/ diff
                    EKg
                    lytes
                    PT, PTT
                    X-ray

    2. Consults   cardiology to discuss pacer

3. Further medical therapy

?HTN - on meds ?

INTRAOP

1. Special considerations

2. Monitors

3. Induction

4. Maintenance

5. Emergence

Preparing for the Anesthesia Orals

6. Intraop problems

Sample Questions

POSTOP

   1. Somnolence

   2. Pulmonary edema

   3. Patient still can't move his legs 4 hours later

Preparing for the Anesthesia Orals

PREOP

1. Labs

ECG: check for the usual problems (MI, rhythm abnormalities) and look for signs of pacemaker dysfunction (pacing spikes that don't capture). If you cannot evaluate the pacer from the ECG, you can have a monitor strip done while the patient is put through maneuvers (Valsalva, squatting) that will increase vagal tone and decrease the heart rate enough to allow the pacer to fire.

Chest x-ray: Check pacer position and whether the lead wires are broken or misplaced.

Sodium: Check the baseline sodium. Hyponatremia is a major concern during a TURP.   *PT, PTT*

2. Consults   A cardiology consult to discuss the specifics of the pacemaker may help. Your *specific* questions to our cardiologic brethren are:

1. What were the indications for the pacemaker?
2. What kind of pacemaker is it?
3. When was the battery last changed?
4. If the pacemaker malfunctions, will placing a magnet over it help or hurt?
5. Is there any sign of pacemaker malfunction?
6. If we have trouble with the pacemaker intraoperatively and can't reprogram it, will you be available with one of those reprogramming briefcases?

3. Further medical therapy   If the pacer is malfunctioning, replace the battery or fix the pacer before the TURP is done. By the way, did we say vital signs are vital? Does that ring a bell? Are you surprised that they are all normal? Wake up and smell the coffee. The pulse is 64. The pacer should probably be firing!

INTRAOP

1. Special considerations   The care and feeding of a pacemaker requires a delicate touch:

1. Keep the grounding pad away from the pacemaker.
2. Use a bipolar Bovey.
3. Use short bursts of the Bovey.

4. Stop the Bovey if the electrical interference with pacer function is adversely affecting hemodynamic stability.

2. Monitors   Use an arterial line or pulse oximeter to correlate QRS complexes with pulsations. You may detect pacemaker malfunction during electrocautery with this monitoring technique.

An arterial line will prove useful for checking serial sodium values.

3. Induction   Barring any contraindication to a regional technique (aortic stenosis with a high gradient, for example), a spinal ought to do the trick. Having the patient awake allows ongoing assessment of mental status.

4. Maintenance   Sedation during the spinal is guided by the patient's age and health. Giving the standard 2 cc of fentanyl and a "few" milligrams of midazolam may cause a respiratory arrest. Small doses of diphenhydramine are good for sedating older patients.

5. Emergence   No specific concerns.

6. Intraop problems

a. *Mental status changes: Do not sedate agitation here* or you fail, period. Think hyponatremia. Check your ABCs, give supplemental oxygen (novel suggestion, huh?), then fire off a sodium. Second on the differential list is hypoxemia from fluid overload and pulmonary edema. Inform the surgeon that his time is limited (continuing dissection will allow more fluid absorption and so lower the sodium). If hyponatremia is indeed the cause of the mental status changes, treat with furosemide and normal saline if the urine output is very brisk. Unless convulsions occur, treatment with hypertonic saline is not needed. When a patient becomes hyponatremic during a TURP, the problem is *excess* body water, not a *lack* of sodium. Thus, treatment is aimed at removing the excess free water rather than adding sodium.

b. *Shoulder pain:* This represents pain referred from the diaphragm. The bladder has ruptured and irrigating fluid is entering the abdomen and irritating the diaphragm. Immediate exploration is mandatory.

c. *Pacemaker malfunction:* Stop the electrocautery. Make sure the grounding pad is far from the pacemaker. Use a bipolar Bovey (they usually use such a unit during a TURP). If the pacer really weirds out, place a magnet over it—that should convert the pacemaker to the V00 (ventricular paced, no chamber sensed, asynchronous firing) mode at a rate of 70 and should at least keep the patient alive until the cardiologist can reprogram the unit. Unfortunately, that maneuver with the magnet doesn't always work, and with the newer programmable models it may actually reprogram the pacemaker to almost anything.

If worse comes to worst and you have to defibrillate the patient, then defibrillate the patient. The discharge may cause an endocardial burn, but ventricular fibrillation causes death.

Cardiologists are usually in house, so go ahead and call one if you are really stuck. They should be able to reprogram a pacemaker gone berserk.

POSTOP

1. Somnolence   A mental status change requires a full court press. First, as always, ABC, ABC, ABC. This somnolence is most likely from:

- *Drugs*—no. 1 cause, excessive sedation
- *Neurologic*—no. 1, syncope from pacer malfunction
- *Metabolic*—no. 1, hyponatremia or hypoxemia

After ABC and stating the simple differential above, go through the complete list.

2. Pulmonary edema   All that absorbed fluid had to go somewhere. This 79-year-old man may very well not have the myocardial oomph to keep the fluid out of his lungs. The amount of absorption from the irrigant (and that irrigation continues postop) is up to 20 mL per minute. Over several hours that adds up. Treatment consists of furosemide, limiting the absorption if at all possible (lowering the bottles of irrigant), sitting the patient up, giving nitroglycerin IV, and providing inotropic support. If this occurs intraop, you should stop the operation, in addition to providing supportive therapy.

3. Patient still can't move his legs 4 hours later   If you used epinephrine in the spinal, the motor block may last a distressingly long time. Before you attribute the long block to epinephrine, though, check for signs of more sinister things, such as an epidural hematoma (pain in the back, variable sensory and motor loss).

In the large blanks now appearing in the questions, we are thinking up likely problems. You may, of course, think of any of a number of other problems.

CASE 17 *(word/phrase approach)*

A 15-year-old, 80 kg boy presents with a suspected fracture and dislocation of his cervical spine from a diving accident. A posterior cervical spine fusion is planned. BP 72/40; P 60; T 37.5°C.

C-spine fracture

C-spine series

Fx what level — ? transection of cord

BP 72/40

spinal cord lesion

C-spine fracture   You are faced with the classic dilemma of securing the airway without damaging the spinal cord. Awake fiberoptic intubation with a pre- and post-intubation neurologic exam is the order of the day. If that fails, an awake tracheotomy is not unreasonable.

On this question you are sure to field the following: "What is the innervation of the larynx?"

Superior laryngeal: sensation above the cords and motor to the cricothyroid

Recurrent laryngeal: intrinsic muscles of the larynx except for the cricothyroid

Which method of topicalization will you use: all topical through the fiberoptic, superior laryngeal block through the mouth or through the skin, transtracheal? Any of these methods is acceptable. Most important is protection of the C-spine. If the topicalization is inadequate and the patient coughs violently on the endotracheal tube, the neurologic injury may worsen. Which method prevents the patient from coughing at all? None—they all make the patient cough at some point. As mentioned in earlier cases, don't say you'll do a block if you don't really know how to do it. Do not volunteer ignorance.

What do you do if (God forbid) a new neurologic lesion does appear despite your best efforts? (that would fit into the *adaptability* part of the exam). Since this case is an emergency, you must proceed. Document the neurologic loss, then provide supportive care: keep oxygenation and acid-base status normal and keep the blood pressure at normal or above normal levels. (There, we did it again, we told you to avoid hypotension and hypoxia.)

What if a new neurologic lesion appeared and the case were elective? Delay the elective case to allow resolution of the injury if surgery is not expected to ameliorate the new injury. This prevents confusing the differential postoperatively. Obtaining the opinion of an expert neurologist before proceeding is always a good idea if time permits.

What would you do differently if the patient had a full stomach? Here *judgment* is important. You must weigh the risk of a C-spine injury against aspiration risks, and come out in favor of protecting the C-spine. Administration of a nonparticulate antacid, ranitidine, and metoclopramide would be our approach since you cannot protect the airway from aspiration at the same time as obliterating movement and coughing with intubation. Once again, imagine yourself in one of your ORs before answering. Then you won't say you would give cricoid pressure if the boy is in a cervical collar.

BP 72/40 Are you really going to attribute that blood pressure to an intracranial or spinal lesion? Look elsewhere—for a ruptured spleen or a pneumothorax, for example. What do you suggest? A chest x-ray will show if there is a pneumothorax. A widened mediastinum suggests a deceleration injury. Do an abdominal exam to see if something is ruptured. Remember, trauma means associated injuries! The patient may be in spinal shock, but that is seen most often with a through-the-cord injury. If this patient's neurologic exam is normal, then spinal shock is most certainly *not* the cause of his hypotension.

spinal cord lesion The examiners can take you one step further and say, "OK, now let's say the patient has a complete section at C6. What does that do to your plan?" ABC, ABC, ABC. With a lesion that high, respiratory compromise may force you to secure the airway right off the bat. You still can't afford to be cavalier, however, since the patient may recover some spinal cord function after the edema of injury wears off. Early in the course of the lesion, spinal shock is a consideration. Later complications include spasticity, autonomic hyperreflexia (uncontrolled reflex outpouring of sympathetic tone, seen in patients with lesions of T7 or higher), and hyperkalemic responses to succinylcholine (starting about 24 hours after injury and continuing for an undetermined time).

All these early and late complications may enter the discussion as the examiners take you from pillar to post on the spinal cord patient.

Hang tough. Three to go.

CASE 18 *(preop/intraop/postop approach)*

A 45-year-old, 60 kg female with 10-year history of myasthenia gravis is admitted for total abdominal hysterectomy (TAH). She has a 50 pack-year history of smoking, and has had multiple episodes of respiratory insufficiency. She is taking pyridostigmine, 60 mg qid, and steroids. BP 100/70; P 70; R 26; vital capacity (VC) 1.4 L.

PREOP

Preparing for the Anesthesia Orals

INTRAOP

Sample Questions

POSTOP

Don't cheat. Work on it yourself before you look.

Preparing for the Anesthesia Orals

PREOP

1. Labs PFTs *à la* FVC, FEV_1, $MMEF_{25-75}$, and a room air blood gas. The main concern here is respiratory. The one value given (vital capacity of 1.4 liters) indicates poor respiratory function. The patient will probably require postoperative ventilation. Be prepared to answer what other values indicate a probable need for postoperative ventilation: concomitant chronic obstructive pulmonary disease (COPD), FVC <2.9 liters, disease lasting more than 6 years, and a pyridostigmine dosage above 750 mg/day. Although small airways disease is not a prominent part of myasthenia gravis, you suspect reactive airways disease from the smoking history, so check for improvement in PFTs on bronchodilator therapy. Any optimization of pulmonary function will help.

2. Consults Even if you know myasthenia well, you should get a neurology consult. A good question for them is, "I am concerned about the patient's respiratory status. Is her dose of anticholinesterase optimal with respect to her respiratory function?"

3. Further medical therapy The only additional therapy would be guided by the neurologist's suggestion. Sometimes plasmapheresis is indicated.

INTRAOP

1. Special considerations *Myasthenia gravis:* By an unknown mechanism (possibly autoimmune), the musculature of myasthenics becomes weak. In effect, the muscles have neuromuscular blockade present.

"Your approach to muscle relaxants, Doctor?" Maybe the relaxant from the inhaled agents alone will do. Any neuromuscular blocker at all may result in prolonged blockade. Use the blockade monitor. Succinylcholine? Maybe it gives a prolonged blockade secondary to pyridostigmine inhibition of cholinesterases; maybe these patients are actually resistant to succinylcholine secondary to blocked receptors, maybe not. Avoid succinylcholine to prevent confusion.

The need for pyridostigmine will not be constant in the perioperative period and may be significantly different from the preoperative requirements.

2. Monitors A-line for frequent blood gas determinations. Although you may not need so many blood gases intraoperatively, you will need them postoperatively as you try to wean the patient.

Sample Questions

Use a neuromuscular monitor. The examiners will *not* assume that you use this monitor unless you say so.

3. Induction   Since the patient is already weak, you should be able to intubate without relaxants. A pentothal/inhaled agent/intubation sequence would work. Cricoid pressure during the induction would be appropriate. The weakness in myasthenics involves the bulbar musculature, so the patient may be at risk for aspiration.

4. Maintenance   Isoflurane provides the most muscle relaxation, therefore it would be a good choice for an inhaled agent. Depending on the blood gases, nitrous oxide is OK. Narcotic supplementation is tempered by a concern for postoperative respiratory depression. This patient has poor baseline respiratory function already, so the least amount of postop respiratory depression is unacceptable.

5. Emergence   At the end of the operation the main concern is, will you extubate the patient? There is no burning need to extubate a patient after a hysterectomy, so at the least sign of respiratory insufficiency, keep the patient intubated.

6. Intraop problems

a. *Bradycardia.* Check ABC. Hypoxia doesn't cause bradycardia right away, but you cannot afford to forget about hypoxia, ever. The most likely cause of bradycardia in an abdominal case is mesenteric traction causing vagal stimulation. Inform the surgeons to cool it.

b. *Tight abdomen.* This is unlikely in a patient with myasthenia, but if the surgeon complains that the musculature is too tight, increase the anesthetic depth or titrate in muscle relaxant with your blockade monitor.

POSTOP

1. Pain   Pain relief is a sticky wicket here. Certainly the patient will be uncomfortable from a hysterectomy, but you don't want to depress respirations. On the other hand, an abdominal operation and pain on inspiration won't help her respiratory function. An epidural infusion of local anesthetic is good, providing pain relief without respiratory depression. Giving intrathecal or epidural narcotics to a patient with such tenuous respiratory status is possible but requires close respiratory monitoring. No matter what the patient gets for pain relief, ICU monitoring is mandatory.

2. Respiratory insufficiency   If the patient does not meet extubation criteria in the immediate postoperative period, only when the environmental milieu is perfect will you be able to attempt extubation. Optimize all the metabolic factors (temperature, potassium, acid-base status, nutrition, magnesium, phosphate), then build up the patient's strength slowly. Work with the neurologist to determine the best dose of an anticholinesterase (too much can put you in a cholinergic crisis with resultant weakness).

CASE 19 *(word/phrase approach)*

A 5-hour-old, 2500 gm infant is scheduled for emergency repair of a congenital diaphragmatic hernia. P 175; R 54; T 35°C; Hgb 12.

Entirely on your own now.

premier push for ① Intracran hem
② immature lungs

ASSOCIATED Anomalies

~~~~~~~~~~~~~~~

5 hours old   Zowie, Batman, the Riddler and the Joker combined couldn't make up a harder question! Go from head to toe on this little rascal. "Well, Dr. Examiner, my concerns in this little tyke include:

head   Premature babies are prone to intraventricular hemorrhage and retrolental fibroplasia. These patients are sensitive to any centrally acting drug such as morphine. The blood-brain barrier is immature, so any centrally acting drug may have increased potency.

What drugs will you use to anesthetize this child? Any inhaled agent may depress the myocardium too much in a premature baby. Nitrous oxide is not acceptable since the patient has abdominal viscera in his chest. Ketamine and/or fentanyl combined with a relaxant is a reasonable choice. You are committed to postoperative ventilation anyway and you can't afford to depress the myocardium, so an IV narcotic technique seems the way to go.

There is no absolutely right answer to the question, "How would you anesthetize this patient?" You, as a consultant in anesthesia, can only propose *a* reasonable answer to that question.

airway   Children have a higher and smaller epiglottis than adults.

lungs   With a congenital diaphragmatic hernia, have a *high* index of suspicion for pneumothorax. Definitely *do not* try to inflate the hyopoplastic lung: inflating it may cause a pneumothorax on the good side.

temperature   Due to their large surface area and poor shivering mechanism, children are prone to hypothermia. Hypothermic babies develop acidosis and respiratory depression. Warm the room, warm the fluids, and keep the baby wrapped (in plastic if available).

fluids   A child of this size (small but not as teeny as a lot of really sick preemies) may not have adequate glucose stores, so you will need to supplement glucose. The open chest will lose a lot of fluid under the lights, so a Foley catheter and a quick response to signs of hypovolemia are mandatory. Also, watch for bubbles in the IV tubing. A neonate this young has a patent or probe-patent foramen ovale.

other   A child with one abnormality may have others (esophageal malformation, cardiac problem, and the like).

vital signs   Are these normal for a newborn? No. The respiratory rate is high and temperature is low. The pulse is also elevated. All

Preparing for the Anesthesia Orals

these signs indicate distress—in this case, respiratory distress. Know pediatric vital signs.

Hct This hematocrit is low for a newborn. Because the patient is in distress and the PDA shunt will reduce oxygen delivery, your threshold for transfusing should be low.

Adapting: What will you say if the Hct is 64? Exchange transfusion may be necessary to prevent sludging of the red cells if appropriate hydration does not reduce the hematocrit.

congenital diaphragmatic hernia The bowel in the chest compromises respiration, so you must first decompress the gut by passing an orogastric or nasogastric tube and suctioning out intestinal contents. Next, avoid ventilating by mask so that you do not fill the intestine with air. Intubate the infant awake. Intraoperatively, suspect pneumothorax at the drop of a hat. If anything at all goes wrong (saturation drops, ventilation becomes difficult, blood pressure drops), think pneumothorax. You may place prophylactic chest tubes.

Preoperatively: A preductal (that means right-sided) pulse oximeter and/or arterial catheter is necessary to assess the oxygen saturation of the blood perfusing the brain.

Intraoperatively: To prevent excess shunting through the patent ductus arteriosus, pulmonary artery resistance must be kept low. Avoid cold, light anesthesia, hypoxia, hypercapnia, acidosis. Desaturation may be related to these factors rather than a pneumothorax. Remember, when the patient gets hypoxemic, bradycardia and hypotension will quickly follow. Don't let that distract you. Treat the hypoxemia. Always remember to say you'll quickly ascertain that the patient is indeed receiving 100% oxygen via an appropriately placed airway.

Postoperatively: The abdomen may be scaphoid, and when muscle relaxation wears off it may be very difficult to ventilate the patient. Incomplete closure or continued paralysis is the response to this problem.

CASE 20 *(preop/intraop/postop approach)*

A 32-year-old, 110 kg black woman with cholelithiasis became pregnant before elective cholecystectomy could be performed. Now, at 28 weeks' gestation, she develops right upper quadrant pain and tenderness with a fever that is unresponsive to supportive measures and antibiotics. She is admitted for cholecystectomy. BP 100/60; P 100; R 26; T 39.8°C; Hct 28.

We saved the best for last—bite the bullet. Hang tough.

It's the day of the boards. They have just given you this stem question. You have 10 minutes to organize on the sheet of paper a reasonable outline of the preop, intraop, and postop problems you are likely to encounter with this patient. Good luck!

pre op :
1) obese — Full stomach
2) how far is preg
3)

op — Induce

PREOP

1. Labs

a. *Room air blood gas.* In a patient of this size, with compressed basilar lung segments from the enlarged uterus, the baseline blood gases may reveal hypoxemia. If the patient requires postoperative ventilation, the baseline blood gases will guide your weaning.

b. *Fetal heart rate.* Although not really a lab value, the fetal heart rate is necessary to determine fetal viability before you induce anesthesia. If the fetus is dead, your anesthetic concerns are different. Coagulopathies may develop.

2. Consults   Have an obstetrician aware that the case is going. On the off chance that the patient requires a C-section, you want the obstetricians to be familiar with the patient.

3. Further medical therapy   No further medical treatment is necessary. Ensure good left uterine displacement as the patient is getting settled on the OR table.

INTRAOP

1. Special considerations   Pregnancy coupled with obesity poses respiratory hazards. The functional residual capacity (FRC) is decreased and oxygen consumption is increased, so this patient will rapidly desaturate if the airway is lost. The airway itself may be hard to manage, with redundant soft tissue in the neck, venous engorgement in the airway itself, and the large breasts impeding laryngoscope manipulation.

Fetal well-being is dependent, by and large, on the mother's well-being. The safest place for a fetus at 28 weeks' gestation is right inside of mom. Keep the mother's physiology well tuned and the fetus should be fine. If the fetus shows signs of distress, fix the mother, don't jump right to C-section. A 28-week newborn delivered emergently would have a host of troubles.

The patient is at risk for aspiration due to her size and her pregnancy. A nonparticulate antacid will at least decrease the pH of her stomach contents. Antihistamines and metoclopramide have never been reported to cause birth defects, but we would still avoid them. The general principle in medicating pregnant patients is, don't give any medication unless you absolutely have to. Who knows what subtle effects may occur from in utero exposure to medications?

2. Monitors

a. *A-line for frequent blood gases*. This patient must have optimal ventilatory management to provide optimal uterine blood flow. If the CO_2 gets too low, for example, uterine artery vasoconstriction will occur.

b. *Fetal heart rate*. You can place a fetal heart rate monitor low on the abdomen and keep the straps out of the way of the cholecystectomy incision. Do not let the surgeon (played by the examiner) dissuade you from placing this essential monitor.

Do you need an obstetrician actually in the room? No, an obstetric nurse well versed in interpretation of fetal heart patterns will provide adequate coverage. An obstetrician should be nearby to help out if trouble develops, but the obstetrician does not need to be in the room.

3. Induction

An awake intubation is safest, given the dire consequences of losing the airway. If a nasogastric (NG) tube has been placed, suction as much as you can.

There is always a concern for mutagenesis. The safest approach is to use drugs with a long history of use in pregnancy: pentothal, morphine, succinylcholine, and pancuronium. It should be noted that the fetus is past the critical time of organogenesis, however.

4. Maintenance

Nitrous oxide may or may not cause abortions and may interfere with protein synthesis. Do yourself a favor and avoid nitrous oxide on the exam. Halothane has the longest history of use, so is considered safest from the standpoint of mutagenesis.

5. Emergence

Since the patient was induced with a full stomach, she must be extubated fully awake. Suction the NG tube before extubation.

6. Intraoperative problems

a. *Loss of variability*. So you give the pentothal and the baby loses variability. What do you do? The answer is, nothing. Losing variability is a normal response to anesthesia. Anything more sinister (late decelerations) on the fetal heart rate monitor requires attention. Treat the ABC of the mother first. Inform the surgeon, and call the obstetrician for his input. *Don't jump to C-section*.

b. *Hypotension*. Left uterine displacement, left uterine displacement, left uterine displacement. Fix that first. The placenta has no autoregulation, so you must treat a low blood pressure quickly. If pressors are necessary, use ephedrine: ephedrine raises blood pressure without constricting uterine blood flow.

POSTOP

1. Unexpected ventricular tachycardia   If, for whatever reason, the patient suddenly develops a malignant arrhythmia, check ABC, then move to cardioversion if hemodynamics deteriorate. Fetuses are not harmed by electric current, but they are harmed by prolonged hypotension.

2. New neurologic deficit   Yeah, we know this doesn't follow, but we're fresh out of things to teach you guys on stem questions.) Nothing worse on the face of the planet. If a patient emerges from anesthesia with a brand new, unsuspected neurologic deficit, all you can do is swallow hard, provide supportive care, and move quickly to diagnosis (which will invariably involve a CT). Keep the blood pressure toward the high end of normal to maintain perfusion pressure. If the patient can't protect her airway, keep her intubated. Some patients just happen to have aneurysms and those aneurysms just happen to rupture during another operation.

There you have a batch of stem questions. Blow away the stem question and you will blow away the exam.

Once you have run the gauntlet of the stem question, you will have to run a mini-gauntlet of mini-questions. The examiners will finish up the stem question and then move on to two or three questions pertaining to different situations.

You will hear something like, "OK, now let's move on to another patient. Say you have a 45-year-old woman post-hysterectomy who now has a urine output of 10 mL/hr."

What follows is a list of such questions. In this part of the test, you need mention only one or two points pertinent to each question. Your answers will be much less involved than in the stem question part of the test.

For this section, we provide only questions. If you have done your homework, you should be able to provide the answers.

1. During a tumultuous labor, a 23-year-old multip suddenly becomes cyanotic and loses consciousness. What is your leading diagnosis, and what steps do you take?

2. During a routine appendectomy, a 9-year-old child's temperature rises from 37.8 to 38.5°C over the course of 30 minutes. What are your next actions?

3. Twenty minutes after a bronchoscopy for peanut aspiration, a 12-year-old child develops stridor. What is your differential diagnosis, and how will you evaluate?

4. One year after a gunshot wound to the hand, a patient is referred to you for management of chronic pain. How do you evaluate this patient?

5. Two weeks after a cholecystectomy, a patient develops jaundice. The internist says that the patient has developed Forane hepatitis. How do you respond? (Hurling epithets and curses back and forth does not constitute an answer.)

6. A pre-eclamptic patient is on magnesium. The newborn appears floppy. What do you do?

7. Which is better for cardiopulmonary resuscitation, epinephrine or norepinephrine? (Oh really? Are you sure? Who says you can't use norepinephrine?)

8. You perform a stellate ganglion block and the patient becomes diaphoretic. What happened?

9. Before an aortic aneurysmectomy a patient has a K$^+$ of 3.1. Do you cancel?

10. A surgeon asks you for preoperative recommendations on a patient with pheochromocytoma. What do you tell him?

11. You are setting up an outpatient surgery clinic and the head nurse wants to know what preop labs you want on the patients. What do you say?

12. A student nurse wants to be a scrub nurse when she finishes school, but she is concerned about the effect of OR pollution on her future pregnancies. What is your advice?

13. What special concerns attend an operation in which lasers are used?

14. A patient presents for emergency replacement of severed digits. He has taken some "nerve pill" for being "bummed out." How does this affect your anesthetic plan?

15. A 72-year-old man is scheduled for a TURP. On exam he has a loud systolic murmur. Is further workup required?

16. The next case in the OB suite is a twin delivery. Your resident asks you if she needs to do anything special for this case. What do you say?

17. You are asked to provide anesthesia for electroconvulsive therapy for a suicidally depressed man. He had an MI last week. Will you do the ECT? What precautions will you take if you decide to proceed?

18. After a retrobulbar block, a patient stops talking to you and becomes dusky. What are your next steps?

19. An 18-year-old primigravida at term has rales, dyspnea, and a loud cardiac murmur. What further workup is required? Suppose she has mitral valve disease, is scheduled for a C-section, and insists on being awake for the delivery. What do you tell her?

20. A 60-year-old man with pancreatic carcinoma is referred for a nerve block. Which block is appropriate?

21. A 10-year-old mentally retarded child must undergo debridement for extensive burns. The surgeon suggests ketamine as usual for his burn patients. How do you respond?

22. A 55-year-old man with chronic obstructive pulmonary disease has been on the ventilator for 2 weeks after a colectomy. You are asked to assist in weaning the patient from the ventilator. What is your protocol?

23. You are asked to develop discharge criteria for an outpatient surgery clinic. What criteria will you recommend?

24. A man with a complete section at T4 presents for cystoscopy. The surgeon suggests that you stand by since the patient can't feel anything, and the surgeon has done several of these under local already. What is your response?

25. A Harrington rod operation is planned. The surgeon wants to know whether a wake-up test, somatosensory evoked potentials, both, or neither is best.

26. A routine cholecystectomy in an otherwise healthy woman turns into a bloody mess. The surgeon reports uncontrollable hemorrhage. The blood bank has only a type and screen. What do you do?

27. An obese man undergoes a hernia repair without incident. The surgeon insists that you extubate deep to avoid coughing. Do you extubate deep to protect the repair?

28. You are called as witness in the case of a man with an ischemic hand following the placement of an arterial line. No Allen test is available in the chart. The plaintiff claims negligence. The courtroom falls silent. All eyes turn to you, the expert. You straighten out your polyester tie, clear your throat, and say . . . .

29. A patient in the ER is thrashing around on the bed after an auto accident. No C-spine film is available yet. He has aspirated and is gasping.

30. A 60-year-old man with longstanding ankylosing spondylitis has just aspirated a safety pin after taking an overdose of tricyclic antidepressants. His chest still hurts from yesterday's myocardial infarction. How do you proceed?

23 | GRAB BAG ANSWERS

Freaked out? Here's a list of clues for the preceding questions. We were just pulling your leg when we said we wouldn't provide answers. The board examiners will be yanking your chain too, but they won't be kidding.

These answers concentrate on the most likely diagnosis and follow-up supportive measures. The examiners will not have the time to take you to the nth degree on these questions.

Once again, you would be well advised to jot down complete answers to the Chapter 22 questions before reading Chapter 23. It's for your own good.

1. Ensure left uterine displacement, provide supplemental O_2, intubate if necessary, and go with full-scale CPR all the way to delivering the baby emergently. Amniotic fluid embolus or thrombotic pulmonary embolus is the most likely diagnosis.

2. Don't go overboard and zip right to Malignant Hyperthermia Land. Heavy drapes, hot lights, or a warm room could contribute to the elevated temperature. If the child shows other signs of MH (tachycardia, increased end-tidal CO_2, tachypnea), then of course send a blood gas and follow the MH guidelines for treatment.

3. Stridor in the recovery room mandates immediate evaluation by you personally (none of this "I'd ask the nurse to . . ."). Inspection of the airway comes first, along with supplemental oxygen. In this case, inspection shows a tooth in the mouth, knocked out during the bronchoscopy. Stridor could also have been due to blood, emesis, a forgotten mouth pack, or postintubation edema. Post-intubation edema can be treated by racemic epinephrine, supplemental humidified oxygen, and reintubation if necessary.

4. Just as increased temperature doesn't *automatically* mean MH, so chronic arm pain doesn't *automatically* mean reflex sympathetic dystrophy. First, before doing a stellate ganglion block, rule out other, treatable causes of arm pain: vascular occlusion, compartment syndrome, retained foreign body, carpal tunnel syndrome. After that workup, and after paying attention to any other medical problems—depression, malnutrition,

ethanol abuse—that could contribute to this condition, go to the stellate ganglion block. The examiners want to know that you are a physician consultant, capable of taking in the big picture. They do not want to board certify a regional block technician.

5. A thorough search for another cause of jaundice must precede any condemnation of anesthetic agents. Review perioperative blood product administration and the preoperative hepatitis status. The operation itself involved the biliary tree and so should prompt a search for a treatable cause of the jaundice (retained stone, operative clip misplaced). Isoflurane as a cause of jaundice is reportable but vanishingly rare. More likely would be hepatitis, cytomegalovirus, or perhaps trauma to the liver itself from retraction on it.

6. Before any erudite discussion on differential diagnosis, resuscitate the newborn and *ensure adequacy of ventilation*. If intubation is necessary, so be it. The most likely diagnosis is magnesium causing muscle weakness, which you can treat with time (let it get eliminated while you support ventilation) or calcium (though you may still have to support ventilation). Other causes of respiratory insufficiency in a newborn include narcotics, pentothal (in high dose), inhaled agents (unlikely, as the obstetricians deliver the baby before much inhaled agent is absorbed), hypovolemia, neurologic insult, and intrauterine asphyxiation.

7. This is a classic, "Golly Moses, I've never *read* that you should use norepinephrine in a resuscitation, but maybe, just maybe, it *is* written down somewhere." Well it's not, your first impression was right. Go with that. Epinephrine's alpha effects provide peripheral vasoconstriction to perfuse the heart and brain while the beta effects can coarsen ventricular fibrillation to make it more amenable to defibrillation.

8. Two kinds of complications can occur from injecting with a needle: the needle can go in the wrong place, or the drug injected through the needle may go to the wrong place. With a stellate ganglion block, the needle can enter the lung (pneumothorax) or the injected drug could go intrathecal (high spinal) or intravascular (in the vertebral artery, just a little dab will cause a seizure; in a vein, a larger dose produces toxicity). For treatment, follow ABC. Provide supplemental O_2 and institute mask ventilation if the patient is apneic. Listen to the chest and get a chest x-ray if pneumothorax is suspected. Support the blood pressure with fluid and/or pressors as required.

Preparing for the Anesthesia Orals

9. The incidence of arrhythmias in patients with low potassium is no higher than in patients with normal potassium. Given the large fluid shifts and renal stresses incident to aortic aneurysm surgery, early replacement of potassium and repeated levels intraop would constitute wise practice. The fatal flaw in these "will you cancel" questions is to cancel without good reason. For example, if you said you would cancel, the examiners would ask why? If you respond, "Because we always cancel them!", you lose.

10. Pheochromocytoma patients require a meticulous preoperative preparation. Most important is alpha blockade and volume replacement. If the patient has congestive heart failure, the preoperative work must be done in an ICU. Certain advocates favor alpha-methyltyrosine to biochemically cut off production of the vasoactive agents (epinephrine and norepinephrine) produced by the pheochromocytoma.

11. For basic outpatient preop labs, men over 40 and women over 50 need an ECG. Women need a hematocrit. Anything else is mandated by the patient's history. Lung disease means a chest x-ray; heart disease an ECG; renal disease, hypertension, or diabetes a set of electrolyte values (specifically, glucose and potassium); liver disease an SGOT. Anyone with liver disease severe enough to merit further workup is not a candidate for outpatient surgery.

Most routine labs are overkill. They do not contribute to patient care and are a useless expense.

12. Studies have shown that OR personnel have a higher incidence of spontaneous abortion than non-OR personnel. These studies did not control for such things as stress. Also, the studies were done before scavenging in the OR was instituted. No inhaled anesthetic has been proved to cause birth defects in humans. Some animal studies have shown a tendency toward increased malformations with exposure to anesthetic gases. In general, in a modern OR where effective scavenging techniques are used, the risk to the fetus is small.

13. Most important is awareness of all OR personnel that they must protect their eyes. Signs on the door must warn of the danger of the laser. Everyone must wear appropriate eye gear that includes side guards on the glasses. Mix air in with the inspired gas mixture to reduce fire hazard (recall that nitrous oxide, but not nitrogen, supports combustion). Guard against fire by using a protected endotracheal tube (none is foolproof, but one with reflective tape or, better yet, a dull matte finish is satisfactory) and by inflating the cuff with colored water (methylene blue, so the sur-

geon can see if he has punctured the balloon). Cover the patient's eyes with damp gauze.

14. Find out which "nerve pill" the patient has taken. If the medication turns out to be an MAO inhibitor, then you've got trouble. Since the case is an emergency, you can't take him off the stuff for 2 weeks (a subject of controversy). Avoid indirect-acting vasopressors, as you may get an exaggerated response. As best you can, avoid narcotics, especially meperidine, since the patient can become hemodynamically unstable. Patients on MAO inhibitors may also develop fever and coma with meperidine administration.

If the patient is on tricyclic antidepressants, he may have an exaggerated response to direct-acting pressor agents. All TCAs have some degree of alpha blockade. The combination of TCA, halothane, and pancuronium produces ventricular arrhythmias; therefore avoid that combination.

15. Murmurs need a complete evaluation. That means echocardiography. This patient may have aortic stenosis. If he does, placing a spinal may drop the blood pressure, never to rise again. The murmur may also indicate some other, unsuspected lesion that may bear on perioperative management. For example, the patient may need prophylaxis against subacute bacterial endocarditis if he has a ventricular septal defect or valvular disease. The prophylaxis would have to cover expected bacteremia from the genitourinary tract.

16. For a twin delivery, give a nonparticulate antacid. The first baby may emerge just fine. The second, however, may run into trouble, and you may have to induce general anesthesia right away. Being prepared for general anesthesia means making sure the patient has received an antacid. Also, make sure there is equipment in the room for two neonatal resuscitations, not just one. That involves rolling the little heated basinette in from the next room.

Left uterine displacement is extra important with the extra large uterus.

17. If the psychiatrist *really* believes that the patient *must* have electroconvulsive therapy, then you must proceed. That is, if the psychiatrist really and truly believes that the risk of suicide outweighs the risk of a perioperative myocardial infarction, then you must go ahead. The actual risk will be somewhere between that of a major surgical procedure done 0 to 3 months after an MI (up to 30% reinfarction) and a cataract (extremely low incidence of reinfarction). It is difficult to extrapolate data on

surgical procedures to an ECT. We'd talk *long and hard* with the psychiatrist and a cardiologist before proceeding.

Given that the examiners will force you to take this case, place an arterial line to follow beat-to-beat blood pressure. Pre-oxygenate, induce with methohexital, and have syringes of labetalol and diluted nitroglycerin at hand to treat the abrupt rush of sympathetic tone that occurs with this procedure. Pretreatment with a beta-blocker may be detrimental, as immediately after the shock, before the sympathetic rush, you can get a big parasympathetic outflow. This can be avoided with IV robinul. Esmolol may help control the heart rate once the sympathetic outpouring occurs.

18. As in the earlier complication from a stellate ganglion block, the needle itself could have gone in the wrong space, or the drugs injected through the needle may have gone into the wrong place. While resuscitating (ABC, ABC, ABC) with bag and mask, think of the differential: intravascular injection, intrathecal injection by tracking backward, oculocardiac reflex with asystole. Treatment consists of supporting ventilation, supporting circulation, and instituting CPR if necessary.

19. Depending on what lesion is causing the cardiac failure, the woman may be able to be awake for the delivery. The differential diagnosis of cardiac failure in pregnancy includes pre-eclampsia, emboli, and pre-existing cardiac disease. The patient with mitral disease, for example, may decompensate with the stress of pregnancy. This patient should undergo echocardiography to determine what lesion she has. Once the lesion is known, invasive monitoring may be needed to manage the patient's fluid status.

You must explain to the mother that general anesthesia may be necessary if that is safest for her and the baby. If she has mitral valve stenosis (a likely lesion), a regional technique may be possible, but only with careful, slow titration of anesthetic level and adequate volume replacement. If general anesthesia is performed, a high-dose narcotic technique may be necessary to prevent a potentially fatal tachycardia with intubation. In such a case, the pediatrician/neonatologist would have to be informed and be available to provide ventilatory support to the narcotized child.

20. First investigate treatable causes for the severe pain (dead bowel, superior mesenteric artery occlusion). In all likelihood, this patient has pain from the carcinoma and will benefit from a celiac plexus block. Even if you don't do these blocks, you should be able to describe the landmarks (L1), the purpose of the block (block the sympathetic outflow from the gut

area), and the possible complications (intravascular injection, high spinal, hypotension from sympathectomy, perforating a large vessel or viscus).

21. Inability to cooperate in a patient who has limited venous access presents severe problems. For dressing changes, IM ketamine may suffice, but a thorough airway evaluation is necessary to establish that you can support ventilation if needed. For intraoperative cases, IM ketamine may at least allow you to get some lines in the patient but may not suffice as a total anesthetic. Once lines are secured, intubate without succinylcholine (for fear of hyperkalemia) and replace volume aggressively (open, bleeding surface areas lose volume rapidly).

22. Weaning is not synonymous with PFTs that are satisfactory for extubation. Weaning means getting the patient in optimal shape to *achieve* those PFTs. Control sepsis, treat underlying infections, minimize carbohydrate load, maximize nutritional support, check electrolytes (including phosphate, calcium, and magnesium), make sure the musculoskeletal system of the thorax is intact (i.e., no flail chest), decompress the gut, have the patient sit up, and gradually build up respiratory muscle strength (any number of protocols exist: slowly decrease intermittent mandatory ventilation [IMV]; decrease IMV and keep patient on CPAP a few hours each day; pressure support; and others), optimize clearance of secretions (that may mean a tracheostomy, especially if the patient has a neurologic impairment), and control bronchospasm. Once these are achieved, you can recite the criteria that mean extubation is possible: negative inspiratory force >30 cm H_2O, tidal volume >5 cc/kg, FVC >15 cc/kg, respiratory rate <30, adequate oxygen saturation on 40% inspired oxygen, etc.

23. To be discharged from an outpatient surgery clinic, persons must display street fitness, that is, they should not need any of the help that medical personnel render. Thus:

- The patient's pain should be controlled by oral meds.
- The patient must be free from nausea.
- The patient must be able to take liquids po.
- The patient must void.
- The patient must ambulate.
- The patient must be in the responsible hands of an adult who can get him back for medical treatment if necessary.
- The patient must be given a number to call so he can have questions answered.

24. Lesions at or about T7 are associated with autonomic hyperreflexia. This uncontrolled reflex outpouring of sympathetic tone can cause heart failure or intracranial bleeding. Although the patient may not feel anything below the lesion, surgical manipulation or minor pain—even bladder distention—may still precipitate this mass reflex. Past operations without incident do not guarantee that the present operation will be incident free. General or spinal anesthesia would both be satisfactory options for the patient. Since defining a level is difficult in a patient with a cord lesion, general anesthesia is the preferred method. Other considerations in the spinal cord injured patient are:

- Volume status is difficult to assess.
- Decubiti may be present. These can tunnel subcutaneously for a long way, making spinal anesthesia problematic.

25. Somatosensory evoked potentials test the *posterior* (sensory) columns; the wake-up test assesses whether the *anterior* (motor) columns are intact. At the risk of sounding like wise guys, the best method of testing both is to test both. Most centers will rely on SSEPs, however.

26. Typed and screened blood has a 1/1,000 chance of causing a major transfusion reaction if the patient has not been transfused before. This is not significantly different from the chance of a reaction from typed and cross-matched blood. In this case, the risk of hemorrhagic shock while waiting for a cross match is much greater than the risk of a transfusion reaction. Send for the typed and screened blood.

27. Anyone who needs a rapid sequence induction (full stomach, obese, pregnant) needs an awake extubation. An obese patient has a high oxygen demand and low FRC; thus a lost airway may result in rapid desaturation. A deep extubation in this patient may result in just such a scenario if the airway is lost. Aspiration is another risk. Given all these considerations, a deep extubation is unwise. Generous narcotics or lidocaine may help prevent violent bucking on the tube, so use these to prevent the patient from tearing apart the surgical repair.

28. The Allen test has no value in predicting which patients will get ischemia from an arterial line. Other than that, you can say nothing about the case without further information.

You may disagree with this answer, but we could easily defend it if pressed. Make sure you can defend your answer.

29. First, secure the airway. Assume the patient has an unstable neck, and have the neurosurgeon hold the head firmly in the neutral position. Have a person trained in performing tracheostomies nearby in case you can't secure an airway. Before you start intubation efforts, resuscitate with bag and mask ventilation with cricoid pressure. You don't want to start what will be a difficult intubation with the patient already hypoxic. Although this patient could theoretically have increased intracranial pressure and you would prefer not to intubate awake, the patient is in extremis and needs a secure airway *now!*

30. Just kidding.

24 | A NOTE ON DRESS AND CONDUCT

We have injected this text with a note of levity, but don't make the mistake of taking that attitude into your exam. The examiners are dead serious in their task, and you should be too. Keep your answers short and to the point. You will have plenty of time to yuck it up after you pass.

Just as you should be serious in your demeanor, you should be the same about your dress. Bopping into the examining room in jogging shorts and a tank top will not impress the examiners. Afterward you can frolic naked in the streets, but dress like a banker for the oral board examination.

25 | POST MORTEM

Anyone who saw "Amadeus" remembers what the emperor of Austria always said: "Well, there it is." And so we say at the end of this little jaunt through Boardland, "There it is."

If you think this book alone will get you through the boards, you are sadly mistaken. This is only a guide, a set of clues. Stick your nose in Dorsch & Dorsch, Stoelting, and Miller (Baby to read, Big to reference). *They* have the information you need. Then sit down with a colleague and do practice exams. You don't need the sample questions we gave, you can make them up yourself. Discuss the cases you will do tomorrow in an oral board format. Consider preoperative assessment and optimization, intraoperative anesthetic plan and likely complications, and postoperative management of pain, urine output, and so forth. That will prepare you for the boards.

Take this book for what it is—a preview of a little chat.

GLOSSARY

AAA   Abdominal aortic aneurysm

ABA   American Board of Anesthesiology

ABC   Airway, breathing, circulation

ARDS   Adult respiratory distress syndrome

ASA   American Board of Anesthesiologists

BUN   Blood urea nitrogen

CABG   Coronary artery bypass graft

CHF   Congestive heart failure

$CMRO_2$ Cerebral metabolic rate of oxygen consumption

CNS   Central nervous system

CPAP   Continuous positive airway pressure

COPD   Chronic obstructive pulmonary disease

CPR   Cardiopulmonary resuscitation

CT   Computed tomography

CVP   Central venous pressure

DOCTOR   The anesthesiologist

DT's   Delirium tremens

ECG   Electrocardiogram

ECT   Electroconvulsive therapy

EEG   Electroencephalogram

FEV_1 Forced expiratory volume in 1 second

FHR   Fetal heart rate

FIO_2 Inspired oxygen fraction

FVC   Forced vital capacity

FRC   Functional residual capacity

ICP   Intracranial pressure

ICU   Intensive care unit

IMV   Intermittent mandatory ventilation

IV   Intravenous

LV   Left ventricle

MAC   Minimum alveolar concentration

MAOI   Monoamine oxidase inhibitors

MAP   Mean arterial pressure

MBC   Maximum breathing capacity

MEFR   Maximal expiratory flow rate

MH   Malignant hyperthermia

MI   Myocardial infarction

$MMEF_{25-75}$ Maximal midexpiratory flow - 25 to 75%

MUGA   Multiple uptake gated acquisition scan

NPO   Nothing by mouth

PCA   Patient-controlled analgesia

PDA   Patent ductus arteriosus

PEEP   Positive end-expiratory pressure

$PEFR_{200-1200}$ Peak expiratory flow rate

PFT   Pulmonary function test

PRN   As needed

RA   Rheumatoid arthritis

RIND   Reversible ischemic neurologic deficit

RV   Residual volume

SGOT   Serum glutamic oxaloacetic transaminase

SURGEON   The anesthesiologist's helper

TAH   Total abdominal hysterectomy

TIA   Transient ischemic attack

TLC   Total lung capacity

TURP   Transurethral resection of the prostate

VC   Vital capacity

VP   Ventriculoperitoneal

V/Q   Ventilation/perfusion ratio

V00   Ventricular paced, nonsensed pacemaker

WSTS   We see this sometimes (a common explanation for many events)

INDEX

ABC (airway, breathing, and circulation), 14, 29, 33, 47, 143, 155, 159
see also Airway
Abdominal aortic aneurysm (AAA), 100–104
Adaptability, 1–2
Addisonian crisis, 127–128, 148
Adrenal problems, 91–92
Adult respiratory distress syndrome (ARDS), 128
Agitation
  and elderly, 127
  and hypoxemia, 112
Air embolism, 58
Airway, 14, 29–31, 61, 186
  and asthma, 29, 30
  and cardiac disease, 30
  and children, 168
  and hematoma, 143
  and hydrocephalus, 98, 99
  and local anesthesia overdose, 47
  and obesity, 55, 71, 172, 185
  and pregnancy, 37, 38
  and rheumatoid arthritis, 126–127
  and spinal, 30
Albumin, 51
Alcohol, cross-tolerance, 91
Alcoholism, 85–92
  and hematocrit, 92
  and hypercapnia, 91
  and hypotension, 92
  and hypoxia, 91, 92
  and liver, 89–92
A-line, 83, 92, 111, 118, 127, 163, 173
Allen test, 177, 185
Allergic reaction, 71
Alveolar proteinosis, 83
American Board of Anesthesiology, 2
  practice exam, 9
  refresher courses, 3, 37
Aminophylline, 23, 110, 111
Ammonia levels, 51

Amniotic fluid embolism, 179
Anaphylaxis, 70, 72
Anemia, 91
Aneurysms, 100–104, 174, 176, 181
  and hypertension, 104
  and tachycardia, 104
Angina, 25
Ankle block, 27
Anticholinesterase, 163, 165
Antihistamines, 172
Aortic aneurysm, 100–104, 176, 181
Apgar scores, 42, 132
Apnea, postoperative, 99–100
Application, 1–2
Arterial line, 38, 154, 169, 183
  and ischemia, 177, 185
Ascites, 90–91
Aspiration, 33, 39, 62, 63
  and awake intubation, 72
  and hypoxemia, 33
  and myasthenia gravis, 164
  and obesity, 56, 65, 172, 185
Associated injuries, 33, 57–60, 147, 159
Asthma, 110, 111, 112
  and airway, 29, 30
Atelectasis, 63, 72
Atlanto-occipital subluxation, 125, 126
Atracurium, 90
Atrial fibrillation, 16, 26
  and digoxin, 76
Atropine, 42, 49, 132
Awake intubation, 28, 61
  and aspiration, 72
  fiberoptic, 125
  and liver disease, 90–91
  and obesity, 55, 71, 72
  and obstetric patient, 39, 65, 173
  and pediatric patient, 43–44
Axillary block, 47, 48

Bain circuit, 18, 19, 99
Baroreceptor reflex, 10

Benzodiazepines, 91
Beta-agonists, 73
Beta blockers, 16, 30, 82, 183
Beta inhalation, 83
Bier block, 47, 48
Biliary spasm, 71, 112
Biopsies, 44–45
Bladder rupture, 75, 154
Bleeding time, 36
Blood-brain barrier, 168
Blood gas, 51, 71, 83, 163
    baseline, 23, 56, 90
    room air, 61, 82, 110, 172
Blood pressure, 58
    see also Hypertension; Hypotension
Books, 3–4, 17, 47, 104, 189
Bovey, 153–154
Bradycardia, 13, 16, 49, 59, 82, 142
    and hypoxia, 164
Brain oxygenation, monitoring, 43, 58
    see also Cerebral perfusion pressure
Breathing circuits, 17–22
Bronchodilator, 23, 70, 110, 111
Bronchopleural fistula, 83
Bronchoscopy, 62, 175
Bronchospasm, 16, 63, 84, 112, 113
Bucking, 99, 142
BUN, 59, 60, 70, 75, 126, 139
Burn patients, 177, 184

Caesarian section, 39, 64, 65–66, 131,
    132, 172, 173
Calcium, 66, 180
Calcium channel blockers, 16, 143
Capnogram, 21, 61
Carbon dioxide, 15–16
    absorber, 16
    and anesthesia machine safety, 21
    and carotid endarterectomy, 141–142
Cardiac disease, 25–28, 63
    and airway, 30
    and aneurysm, 103
    and carotid endarterectomy, 26–27,
        140, 142
    and obesity, 56, 71
    and oliguria, 35
    and pregnancy, 37, 183
    and thoracotomy, 77–85
Cardiologist, 25
    consult with, 26, 76, 82, 147, 153
    and pacemaker, 153, 155
Cardiopulmonary resuscitation (CPR),
    47, 58, 176, 179, 183

Carotid bruit, 82
Carotid endarterectomy, 82, 132–143
    and cardiac disease, 26–27, 140, 142
    and hypertension, 140–141
    and hypotension, 142
    and tachycardia, 142
Celiac plexus block, 183–184
Central venous line, 41, 65
    and alcoholism, 92
    and hypovolemia, 127
Central venous pressure (CVP), 61, 72
Cerebral perfusion pressure, 27, 50, 141
Cerebral steal, 141–142
Cervical plexus block, 140
Cervical spine trauma, 33, 147, 156–
    159, 166
    and hypotension, 158, 159
Chest x-ray, 25, 26, 59
    and aspiration, 63
    and pacemaker, 153
    and rheumatoid lung, 126
Children, 41–45
    intubation, 29, 43–44
    see also Pediatrics
Cholestectomy, 30, 52, 66–73, 104–
    113, 170–174
    and jaundice, 175
Chronic cough, 23
Chronic obstructive pulmonary disease
    (COPD), 23, 163, 177, 184
Cimetidine, 65, 111
Circle system, 19
Cirrhotics, 51–52, 89–92
    and halothane, 90
Clarity, 1–2, 26
Coagulation, 90
    parameters, 51
Coding, 85
Computerized axial tomography (CT),
    33, 174
Congenital diaphragmatic hernia, 43–
    44, 166–169
Congestive heart failure, 49, 65
Consults
    cardiology, 26, 76, 82, 147, 153
    neurology, 82, 126, 147
    obstetric, 172
    pediatric, 98
    pulmonary, 82, 110
    radiology, 126
Continuous positive airway pressure
    (CPAP), 84
Cor pulmonale, 56, 71

Preparing for the Anesthesia Orals

Coronary artery bypass graft, 26–27, 29
Coronary steal, 84, 141–142
Craniotomy, 58–59
Creatinine, 70, 75, 126, 139
Cricoid pressure, 55, 111, 159, 164
Cricothyrotomy, 39, 99, 126
Cyanosis, 175

Dantrolene, 3, 44, 45
Decadron, 31
Defibrillator, 76, 155
Delayed awakening, 143
Delayed emergence, 148
Delirium tremens, 91, 92
Dexamethasone, 58
Diabetes, 70–72
Dialysis, 35–36
Digoxin, 16, 76
Diphenhydramine, 72, 154
Dipyridamole-thallium perfusion scan, 26, 27, 139
Dopamine, 35, 70
Double lumen tube, 83, 84, 120
Dress and conduct at exam, 187
Dyspnea, 23, 26

Eaton-Lambert syndrome, 118
Electrical safety and anesthesia machine, 21–22
Electrocardiograph (ECG), 26
   and carotid endarterectomy, 142
   comparison between old and new, 25, 82, 120–121, 126, 139
   and microshock, 22
   and pacemaker dysfunction, 153
   ST segments, 30
Electroconvulsive therapy, 176, 182–183
Electrolytes, 36
Emergence delirium, 91
Endobronchial intubation, 72
Endotracheal tube, 42, 132
   and lasers, 181
   misplaced, 63, 99
End-tidal CO_2, 83, 118, 179
Enflurane/oxygen, 62, 71, 84, 111, 112, 148
Ephedrinate, 33
Ephedrine, 62, 173
Epidural, 27, 37, 48, 62–63, 72
Epidural hematoma, 39, 65, 155
Epiglottis, 41–42

Epinephrine, 42, 58, 72, 131, 132, 155, 179
   and CPR, 176
Esmolol, 84, 183
Esophageal intubation, 16
Etomidate, 111

Failed intubation, 39, 62, 127
Fail-safe mechanism, 19
Femoropopliteal, 27
Fentanyl, 148, 154, 168
Fetal heart rate, 131–132, 172, 173
Fiberoptic bronchoscope, 84
Fiberoptic intubation, 29–30, 71
   awake, 125
Flowmeters, 19, 20
Foley catheter, 61, 63, 71, 83, 127, 168
   kinked, 35
Forane hepatitis, 175
Full stomach, 30–31, 56
   and ascites, 90–91
   and cervical spine injury, 158–159
   and gastric resection, 110–111
   and pediatric patient, 41, 42
   and pregnancy, 37–38
   suctioning, 43
Functional residual capacity (FRC), 90
Furosemide, 35, 58, 75, 154
   and potassium, 139
   and pulmonary edema, 155

Gastric resection, 110–111
Geriatric patients, 58–60
Gestational age, 97, 99–100
GI evaluation, 89
Glucose hemostasis, 51
Glycogen stores, 90

Halothane, 62, 84, 111, 173
   and cirrhotics, 90
   and hepatitis, 52, 62
   and intracranial pressure, 99
Hand ventilation, 20, 33, 84
Hanging bellows, 21
Harrington rod operation, 177, 185
Heart rate control, 76
   fetal, 131–132, 172, 173
   see also Tachycardia
Heat and infants, 98, 168
Hematocrit, 13, 126
   and alcoholism, 92
   and bleeding, 104

and infants, 97, 169
monitoring, 127
and obesity, 56
and transfusion, 53, 97, 148, 169
Hematoma, 143
epidural, 143
Heparin, 26, 76
Hepatitis, 175, 180
and halothane, 52, 62
Hip surgery, 121–128
Hoarseness, 148
Holter monitor, 139, 148
Humerus, fracture of, 144–148
Hydralazine, 84
Hydrocephalus, 92–100
and airway, 98, 99
Hyperalimentation, 60–61, 62
Hypercapnia, 13, 14, 15–16, 70
and alcoholism, 91
and bucking, 99
and intracranial pressure, 98
Hyperkalemia, 75, 159, 184
Hyperpnea, 45
Hypertension, 13, 14
and aneurysm, 104
and carotid endarterectomy, 140–141
and intracranial pressure, 31
and lung cancer, 120
and obesity, 56
and pregnancy, 65
Hyperventilation, 99
Hypoglycemia, 71, 97
and liver disease, 90, 91
Hypokalemia, 43, 59, 181
Hyponatremia, 75, 91, 112, 153, 154, 155
Hypotension, 13, 14, 17–28, 62
and alcoholism, 92
and carotid endarterectomy, 142
and cervical spine trauma, 158, 159
and hypothyroidism, 148
and pregnancy, 37, 131, 173
Hypothyroidism, 148
Hypoventilation, 16
Hypovolemia, 14, 35, 41, 103–104, 131, 148
and pregnancy, 131
Hypoxemia, 13, 14–15, 63, 155
and agitation, 112
and aspiration, 33
and liver disease, 91
and lung deflation, 84

and obesity, 56, 70, 71, 72
and pediatric patients, 44, 169
Hypoxia, 120, 158
and alcoholism, 91, 92
and bradycardia, 164
and intracranial pressure, 31, 98
Hypoxic pulmonary vasoconstriction, 83
Hysterectomy, 160–165

ICU, 72, 75
Interscalene block, 48
Intracranial hemorrhage, 65
Intracranial pressure, 31, 58, 98
and halothane, 99
and hydrocephalus, 98
and hypercapnia, 98
and hypertension, 31
and ketamine, 99
and nitrous oxide, 99
Intrathecal, 62–63, 72
and pregnancy, 38
Intraventricular hemorrhage, 168
Ischemia, 177, 185
Isoflurane, 62, 84, 99, 111, 112, 141, 164, 180
IV insertion, 98

Jackson Reese circuit, 18, 19, 99
Jaundice, 175, 180
Judgment, 1–2

Ketamine, 2, 39, 111, 131, 148, 168
and burn patients, 177, 184
and intracranial pressure, 99
Ketosis, 70, 71
Kidney, 35–36
and aneurysm, 103
and diabetes, 70
and pre-eclampsia, 38
Korsakoff's psychosis, 92
Kyphoscoliosis, 15

Labetalol hydrochloride, 104
Labetolol, 84, 142, 183
Laparotomy, 60–63
Laryngoscopy, 16, 127
Larynx, innervation, 158
Lasers, safety precautions, 176, 181
Lasix, 31
Left uterine displacement, 131, 173, 179, 182
Librium, 91

Lidocaine, 42, 84, 142, 185
  and intubation, 111
Line isolation monitor, 17, 21–22
Liver disease
  and alcoholism, 89–92
  and awake intubation, 90–91
  and rapid sequence induction, 90–91
  tests, 51–52
Lobectomy, 23–24, 82
Lopressor, 104
Lung cancer, 77–85, 113–121

Macroshock, 21
Magnesium, 66, 175, 180
Malignant hyperthermia, 3, 16, 44–45,
    179
  and alcoholism, 90
Malnutrition, 118
Mannitol, 31, 58
Mapleson circuits, 16, 17–18, 19
Masseter spasm, 44, 45
Meperidine, 182
Mepivacaine, 47
Metoclopramide, 56, 65, 111, 158, 172
Metoprolol, 84
Microshock, 22
Midazolam, 154
Minoxidil, 164
Mitral valve stenosis, 183
Monoamine oxidase inhibition (MAOI),
    182
Morphine, 143, 168, 173
MUGA, 24, 26, 121
Murmurs, 176, 182, 183
Muscle relaxants, 163
Myasthenia gravis, 160–165
Myocardial infarction, 75–76
  and electroconvulsive therapy, 176,
    182–183
  perioperative reinfarction rate, 74
  postop mortality, 75
  tests for, 26
  and thoracotomy, 77

Naloxone, 112
Narcan, 143
Narcotics, 16
Nasal fiberoptic, 126
Nasogastric tube, 61
Neonatal resuscitation, 42
Neurology consult, 82, 126, 147

Neuromuscular block, 16, 90, 91, 118,
    163
  monitor, 163, 164
Nitrogylcerin, 30, 70, 155, 183
  and biliary spasm, 112
  sublingual, 76, 143
Nitrous oxide, 62, 71, 164, 168
  and abortion, 99
  and anesthesia machine safety, 19
  and intracranial pressure, 99
Nontriggering anesthetic, 44, 45
Norepinephrine, 176, 180

Obesity, 55–56, 70–73
  and airway, 55, 71, 172, 185
  and aspiration, 56, 65, 172, 185
  and awake intubation, 55, 71, 72
  and cardiac disease, 56, 71
  and hematocrit, 56
  and hypertension, 56
  and hypoxemia, 56, 70, 71, 72
  and pain, 72
  and pregnancy, 65, 172
  and pulmonary function test, 55–56,
    70
  and rapid sequence induction, 55–56,
    65
Obstetrics, 37–39, 166–169, 183
  and awake intubation, 39, 65, 173
  consult, 172
  and spinal, 39
Oculocardiac reflex, 11, 16, 49, 183
Oliguria, 35–36, 38, 65, 66
  and cardiac disease, 35
Open eye, 29, 30–31, 49
Outpatient surgery clinic
  discharge criteria, 177, 184
  preop labs, 176, 181
Oxygen and anesthetic machine safety,
    19–20
Oxygen saturation dropping, 99

Pacemaker, 149–155
Pain, 62–63
  and hypertension, 14
  and hysterectomy, 164
  and obesity, 72
Pancreatic carcinoma block, 177, 183–
    184
Pancuronium, 111, 173
  and transient ischemic attack, 182
Patent ductus arteriosus (PDA), 44

Patient controlled analgesia (PCA), 62–63

Pediatrics, 41–45, 92–100
  and awake intubation, 43–44
  consult, 98
  and full stomach, 41, 42
  and hypoxemia, 44, 169
  and pneumothorax, 44, 168, 169
  and rapid sequence induction, 43

PEEP, 63, 72, 84, 120
Pelvic pain, 131
Pentothal, 31, 47, 99, 111, 141, 148, 164, 173
Peritoneum, traction on, 16
Phenylephrine, 131
Pheochromocytoma, 176, 181
Pickwickian patient, 56, 70, 71
Placenta previa, 131
Placental abruption, 131
Platelet dysfunction, 36, 38, 39, 65
  and liver disease, 90
Pneumonectomy, 23–24, 82, 118–120
Pneumothorax, 48, 63, 72, 113, 154
  and children, 44, 168, 169
  tension, 33, 147
Post-intubation edema, 179
Pre-eclampsia, 38–39, 65–66, 175, 180, 183
Pregnancy
  and airway, 37, 38
  and cardiac disease, 37, 183
  and full stomach, 37–38
  and hypertension, 65
  and hypotension, 37, 131, 173
  and hypovolemia, 131
  normal physiology of, 37–38
  and obesity, 65, 172
  and OR nurses, 176, 181
Premature babies, 168
Preoxygenation, 56, 65
Pressors, 27
Procaine, 71
Prostate. *See* Transurethral resection of the prostate (TURP)
Protein-bound drugs, 90, 118
Proteinuria, 38, 65
Pulmonary artery catheter, 38, 65, 83, 121
  and embolism, 128
  and liver disease, 92
Pulmonary edema, 65, 155
Pulmonary embolism, 128

Pulmonary function test (PFT), 3, 23–24, 82, 163
  and asthma, 110
  and lung cancer, 118
  and obesity, 55–56, 70
  and ventilator, weaning from, 184
Pulse oximeter, 154
Purulence and lung, 83
Pyloric stenosis, 43
Pyridostigmine, 163

Q waves, 120–121

Radiology consult, 126
Ranitidine, 56, 65, 158
Rapid sequence induction, 41, 61, 71, 185
  and emergency assumption, 103
  and liver disease, 90–91
  and obesity, 55–56, 65
  and pediatric patients, 43
Recommended reading, 3–4, 17, 189
Reflex sympathetic dystrophy, 179
Regional anesthetics, 48
  and asthma, 30
  and carotid endarterectomy, 141
  and hip surgery, 126, 127
  and nausea, 142
  and vaginal bleeding, 131
Reservoir bag, 20
Retrobulbar block, 176, 183
Retrolental fibroplasia, 43, 98, 168
Reversible ischemic neurological deficit (RIND), 27
Rheumatoid arthritis, 121–128
Robinul, 183
Room air blood gas, 61, 82, 110, 172

Safety factors of anesthesia machine, 19–22
Scavenging system, 20, 181
SGOT, 51–52, 61, 89
Silent ischemia, 27, 70
Smokers, 60–63, 118, 160–165
Sodium concentration, 51, 153, 154
Somatosensory evoked potentials, 177, 185
Somnolence, 155
Spinal, 48, 75, 127, 185
  and airway, 30
  and obstetric patient, 39
  sedation and age of patient, 159

Preparing for the Anesthesia Orals

Split lung function studies, 118–120
Steal, 84, 141–142
Stellate ganglion block, 176, 179, 180, 183
Steroids, 72, 127–128, 148
Stridor, 100, 175, 179
Stroke, perioperative mortality
Subdural hematoma, 92
Succinylcholine, 31, 45, 47, 159, 163, 173
  and hyperkalemia, 184
Supine hypotension syndrome, 37
Swan catheter, 11, 41, 76
Syncopal episode, 57, 58, 147

Tachycardia, 13, 27–28, 30, 45, 76, 80, 174
  and aneurysm, 104
  and bronchodilators, 111
  and carotid endarterectomy, 142
  fetal, 131
  primary, 14
  secondary, 14
  treatment, 83
Temperature, 148, 168
Tension pneumothorax, 33, 147
Textbooks of anesthesiology, 3
Theophylline level, 83, 110
Thiamine, 91
Thoractomy, 77–85, 118–120
  and cardiac disease, 77–85
Thrombocytenia, 53
Thyroid dysfunction, 2, 148
  and alcoholism, 92
  see also Hypothyroidism
Thyrotoxicosis, 16
Tight abdomen, 164
Tonsil, bleeding, 41
Total body water, 90
Toxicity, 47–48
Tracheostomy, 39, 41–42, 55, 186
Transfusion, 53–54
  and alcoholism, 92
  and hematocrit, 53, 97, 148, 169

and infant, 97, 169
  reaction to, 177, 185
Transient ischemic attack, 27, 139, 140
  and halothane, 182
Transient syncopal episode, 57, 58
Transurethral resection of the prostate (TURP), 73–76, 149–155, 176, 182
Trauma, 2
  and associated injuries, 33, 57–60, 147, 159
Trendelenburg position, 27, 33, 62, 127
Tricyclic antidepressants, 182
Twins, delivery of, 182
Tylenol, 59

Ultrasound, 131
Urinary obstruction, 75
Urine output, 35–36, 63, 97–98
  see also Oliguria
Uterine hypertonus, 13

Vagal stimulation, 16, 30, 164
Vaginal bleeding, 137
Vaporizers, 17
Vecuronium, 31, 99, 111
Ventilator, weaning from, 73, 172, 177, 184
Ventricular dysfunction, 121
Ventricular fibrillation, 76
  and microshock, 22
Ventricular peritoneal shunt, 92–100
Verpamil, 84
Vital signs, 13–16, 59, 76
  and age of patient, 42
Vitamin K, 91
Vomiting, 57–58

Warfarin, 76

X-ray
  cervical spine, 125
  chest, 25, 26, 59, 63, 96, 126, 153